Pilot's Operating Handbook for Health

Pilot's Operating Handbook for Health

**PREVENTIVE MAINTENANCE FOR YOUR HEART OR
HOW TO STAY IN THE LEFT SEAT FOR LIFE**

By a Pilot for Pilots

Jacqueline Brunetti, MD
Senior Aviation Medical Examiner

Copyright © 2016 Jacqueline Brunetti, MD
All rights reserved.

ISBN: 1523730692
ISBN 13: 9781523730698
Library of Congress Control Number: 2016901560
CreateSpace Independent Publishing Platform
North Charleston, South Carolina

*This book is dedicated to
all who fly with the eagles.*

Contents

Preface ix

Introduction xiii

Chapter 1 Why Are All These People Sick? 1

Chapter 2 Systems and Descriptions 5

Chapter 3 Human Factors 14

Chapter 4 Recommendations for Health 25

Chapter 5 Hazard Avoidance 51

Chapter 6 Annual Inspection—What Is Your Risk of
           Heart Disease? 64

Chapter 7 Conclusion 83

Checklist · 87

Recommendations · 89

About The Author · 93

Notes · 95

Preface

There are very few professions that require periodic medical examination and clearance to allow continued employment. Probably only a small percentage of people sitting in the rows behind the cockpit of a commercial airliner is aware that airline pilots are evaluated every six months by a Federal Aviation Administration (FAA) designated aviation medical examiner (AME) to determine "fitness to fly." This is mandated by the FAA to ensure the safety of the flying public. Consequently, preservation of health becomes a key issue for airline pilots, as continued employment will depend on maintaining valid medical certificates.

There are three medical-certificate classes that can be issued by an AME, a physician instructed by the FAA in aviation medical standards and also required to undergo periodic retraining at three-year intervals:

Class 1: Airline-transport pilots

Class 2: Commercial pilots, flight engineers, flight navigators, air-traffic controllers

Class 3: Private pilots, recreational pilots, student pilots

The FAA has developed a list of medical standards for each class that must be met by the airman, and there is a list of diagnoses that result in denial of certification. The disqualifying medical conditions are listed below in alphabetical order.

1. Angina pectoris
2. Bipolar disorder
3. Cardiac valve replacement
4. Coronary heart disease that has required treatment or, if untreated, has been symptomatic or clinically significant
5. Diabetes mellitus requiring insulin or other hypoglycemic medication
6. Disturbance of consciousness without satisfactory medical explanation of the cause
7. Epilepsy
8. Heart transplant
9. Myocardial infarction
10. Permanent cardiac pacemaker
11. Personality disorder that is severe enough to have repeatedly manifested itself by overt acts
12. Psychosis
13. Substance abuse and dependence
14. Transient loss of control of nervous-system function(s) without satisfactory medical explanation of cause

An airman who is medically disqualified for any reason may apply for reconsideration by the FAA. This process involves additional documentation and testing that can be costly and time consuming; an official Authorization for Special Issuance of a Medical Certificate is granted only if certain parameters specific to each condition can be met.

Of these disqualifying conditions, those related to coronary heart disease—angina, coronary heart disease that has required treatment or is symptomatic, and myocardial infarction—can potentially be prevented, or at least ameliorated, by lifestyle modification. My aim in writing this book is to educate airmen, and anybody else willing to spend the time to read this book, about how coronary heart disease develops. Understanding how a pliable blood vessel can become a narrowed, rigid tube that blocks blood flow and learning what might prevent this cascade of events will hopefully spur the reader to adopt heart-healthy lifestyle changes. As every pilot and non-pilot knows, it is much better to prevent an accident than to deal with the aftermath.

Every airplane is equipped with a pilot-operating handbook (or POH) that explains the operations and limitations of the aircraft as well as recommended maintenance. Every instrument installed in the airplane also has its specific instruction manual. *This book* is an operating manual for the airman, the pilot in command (PIC), who sits in the left seat of the cockpit.

I am confident that an adequate understanding of normal body processes and the mechanisms that promote disease is not beyond the grasp of any person, if presented in plain language. This book attempts to demystify the topic of heart disease. I have chosen this particular topic not only because this condition can result in denial of medical certification for pilots but also because the drivers of heart disease are integrally shared by other chronic disease states, including obesity, diabetes, and cancer. No one in his or her right mind would sit behind the controls of an aircraft without proper training and think that he or she could commandeer a plane without dire consequences. The human body is incredibly resilient, but continued and persistent misuse of a body also has its consequences. The concepts presented in the next pages are not revolutionary—just common sense.

Jacqueline Brunetti, MD

Introduction

> The pleasures of an open mind are greater than the pleasures of thinking you have discovered the truth.
> —E. James Potchen, MD, Distinguished Professor and Chair Emeritus at Michigan State University Department of Radiology

I am a pilot, one of a group of human beings dissatisfied with the grip of gravity and longing to be up in the air. I first considered learning to fly at age seventeen while summering at my grandfather's house on Long Island, when I discovered an advertisement for flight lessons at East Hampton Airport. Growing up in an Italian American family—particularly *my* Italian American family—did not allow a young woman this particular brand of independence. So it wasn't until the age of forty that I earned my wings. I was told at the time that flight was the "last bastion of male dominance." That was particularly appealing to me, as I never thought I needed equality; I wanted to be *better* than the guys.

In order to expand my love of flying into my day job as a physician, I applied for and was accepted into the FAA training program to become an aviation medical examiner in 1994. I have been a senior aviation medical examiner since 2000 and an FAA employee examiner since 2013. Those designations permit me to perform required periodic medical exams not only for general aviation pilots but also for airline pilots, FAA inspectors, and the people behind the scenes in air-traffic control. Because of my own family history, the topic of heart disease—one of the conditions that all airmen know can potentially result in a denial of medical certification (and for a commercial airline pilot, a loss of livelihood)—has been of particular interest to me. I have chosen this as the topic of this book, rather than more common problems such as obesity and type 2 diabetes, because there is a certain "fear factor" associated with the idea of a heart attack, a more potent catalyst for lifestyle change. And in fact, as you will see, the factors underlying heart disease, obesity, and type 2 diabetes are closely related.

Although in medical school and during my internship I found the pathophysiology of heart disease fascinating, the actual practice of cardiology in the 1970s was not to my liking. I discovered that my greatest talent was interpreting a patient's imaging studies. So I turned away from internal medicine, where I felt frustrated by my inability to *cure* patients with chronic disease, and embraced the life of the radiologist, the Sherlock Holmes of the medical field. For more than three decades, I have been the doc in the back room, interpreting the films or scans ordered by your physician. I have professional boards in diagnostic radiology, nuclear medicine, and nuclear radiology, so I am well versed in both anatomic and functional pathophysiology. This profession has given me a unique vantage point in the medical field in that I can both understand and see the effects of illness in all organ systems. I have observed the results—some successful, some not or only temporary—of efforts to stop or reverse disease.

Over the last few decades, as increasing emergency-room visits resulted in increasing numbers of radiological procedures, I was compelled to wonder, "Why are all these people sick?" I remember reading an article in 1994 written by Dr. Clifton Meador in the *New England Journal of Medicine* titled "The Last Well Person." The article was a response to a young physician's comment that "a well person is a patient who has not been completely worked up." Meador comments that while at a dinner party, he realized that everyone there had a diagnosis of some sort, and in fact he had not met a completely well person in months. He writes, "What is paradoxical about our awesome diagnostic power is that we do not have a test to distinguish a well person from a sick one."[1]

Is this so far from reality? I don't think so. Just spend one afternoon in front of your television. It is a never-ending symphony of arthritis, reflux, high cholesterol, constipation, and erectile dysfunction, all with the command to "ask your doctor." With all of this marketing, it is not surprising that illness is accepted as the normal state of being. Is illness normal? Of course not! But the fact is that in the United States and globally, the incidence of obesity, heart disease, and neurodegenerative diseases continues to rise.

The frustration of not knowing the answer to the question "Why are all these people sick?" placed me on yet another path of inquiry. In 2013, I completed Dr. Andrew Weil's two-year distance-learning fellowship in integrative medicine at the University of Arizona. This comprehensive one-thousand-hour program of study provided me with the additional tools I needed to better understand the roles of diet, exercise, stress, and the environment on health and disease. In February 2015, I successfully passed the board exam in integrative medicine. And so I return to the issue at hand: Is heart disease inevitable? Is it possible to prevent, halt, or even reverse heart disease? I am convinced that the answer is yes.

This book is written mainly for pilots but is useful for all who desire to be the captains of their ship and masters of their fate. The idea was planted in my psyche by Dr. Tieraona Low Dog, former director of my integrative medicine fellowship; she's an outstanding teacher, wise woman, author, and current fellowship director of the Academy of Integrative Health and Medicine.

Aging is inevitable, but risk of disease can be modified. I will present in this book the current understanding of the cause of heart and vascular disease as well as strategies to reduce your risk. I will present the science behind the recommendations for heart-disease risk reduction. If you can understand why an airplane flies and what can make it fall out of the sky, there is no reason why understanding human physiology should be out of your reach.

CHAPTER 1

Why Are All These People Sick?

> It's not one thing that kills you. It's a
> series of mistakes that will kill you.
> —Old pilot adage

This book is about heart disease, specifically coronary artery disease, but the fact is that many of the factors responsible for increased heart-disease risk also promote other degenerative illnesses such as liver disease, diabetes, and cancer. Despite millions of dollars spent for research and drug development, heart disease remains the most frequent cause of death worldwide.

In September 2013, United Flight 1603 safely diverted course to Boise, Idaho, on flight from Houston to Seattle after declaring an in-flight emergency when the sixty-three-year-old United Airline captain suffered a fatal heart attack. This event reopened debate regarding public safety, the 2007 FAA decision to raise commercial-pilot retirement age from sixty to sixty-five, and the adequacy of the FAA medical examination in detecting potentially debilitating diseases. In

October 2015, a fifty-seven-year-old American Airlines captain expired midflight between Phoenix and Boston.

Now, taken individually, these events are extremely unnerving for the flying public; however, the risk of in-flight pilot incapacitation is extremely low. A 2012 study in the journal *Aviation Space and Environmental Medicine* reported an annual incapacitation, in the year 2004, of 0.25 percent in commercial pilots in the United Kingdom who hold Class 1 Medical Certificates.[2] Half of these events were related to cardiac or cerebrovascular disease. An older study of general aviation accidents from 1978 reports a less than 1 percent incidence of cardiovascular incapacitation as the primary cause of a fatal aviation accident.[3] Commercial flights always have at least two pilot crews, so these are pretty good odds for the flying public—but what about the pilot? What if you are in the one-quarter of 1 percent? How would you know that you are at risk?

Cardiovascular disease is the result of a combination of factors, most—if not all—of which are modifiable. To me, that means that heart disease is not inevitable. You can change a course that has placed you in the direction of disaster!

You are in some ways like your airplane, and I suspect some of you take better care of your aircrafts than yourselves. Nonetheless, I have known general aviation pilots who gladly accept bargain-priced annual inspections on their airplanes, thinking a four-hundred-dollar job will be just as good as one that rightly costs four thousand dollars! There is no denying the fact that faulty aircraft systems can kill you. But do you understand that malfunctioning body systems can kill you without warning? Let's look at this in aviation terms.

HOBBS Meter: We all have our individually programmed TBO (Time before Engine Overhaul); this is our genetic makeup.

Components wear out, but if carefully flown, an engine can exceed TBO.

Fuel: You can't put piston engine gasoline into a jet engine. You are what you eat!

V_{NE}: (Never exceed speed). Stress can be both a stimulus and a killer. Chronic stress without solution is destructive and potentially fatal.

Annual Inspection: Preventive maintenance and the right testing can keep you flying safely.

Ramp Time: An engine not flown is as dangerous as one that is not serviced. A sedentary lifestyle is as bad as, and maybe worse than, a bad diet.

As every pilot knows, flight planning is critical to safe operations in the airways. The chapters that follow are a "life plan" to help *vector* you away from hazards and toward the goal of a healthy life.

VECTORS FOR CARDIOVASCULAR HEALTH

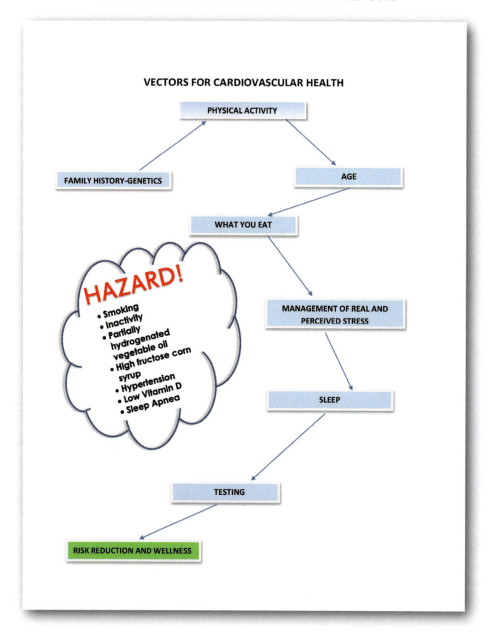

CHAPTER 2

Systems and Descriptions

What makes a normal blood vessel turn into a time bomb? Fats in your bloodstream invade the lining of your coronary arteries. These fats are called plaque. Over a period of time, some of these deposits of plaques continue to increase in size. In an attempt to heal the lesion, the body forms a calcified cap on the plaque. A heart attack happens when the cap breaks down, releasing substances into the vessel that cause a blood clot to form. A clot blocks blood flow from carrying oxygen and nutrients to the heart muscle. If not treated, this results in damage to the heart muscle—a heart attack.

Your heart is your body's fuel pump. It is a unique organ that is programmed to start beating in an embryo about three to four weeks after conception. Controlled by a network of fibers that carry electrical impulses, causing the muscle to contract, the heart continues to perform for multiple decades.

The heart has four chambers separated by valves: two atria that act as passive reservoirs and two ventricles that do the work of moving blood. The right atrium receives blood from the body via veins called the superior and inferior vena cava. The right ventricle delivers blood to the lungs to exchange waste carbon dioxide (CO_2) and water (H_2O) for oxygen (O_2), which is needed for almost every enzymatic function in the body. The left atrium receives the oxygenated blood from the lungs, and the left ventricle propels the blood into the aorta and out to the rest of the body. The heart muscle receives its blood and nutrients via the right and left coronary arteries, which are the first branches of the aorta.

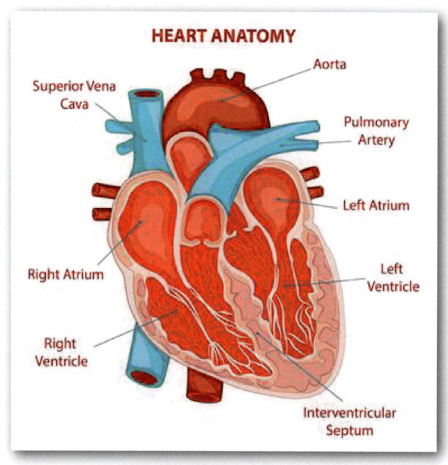

©Okili77/Shutterstock.com

Your coronary arteries, to your body, are the equivalent of the fuel lines to your aircraft. They carry oxygen and nutrients to your engine, the heart muscle.

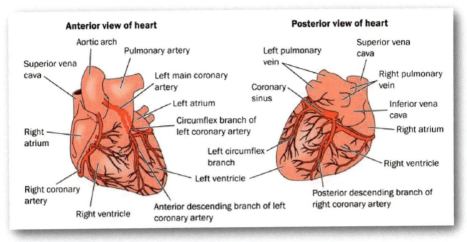

© Legger | Dreamstime.com

These vessels dilate and deliver more blood when there is increased demand or as heart rates go up. The ability for arteries to dilate is critical. When they become rigid and narrowed, as happens with age and atherosclerosis, the result is similar to that of a blocked fuel line. A partially blocked line might result in engine sputter. Or, the engine with a partially blocked fuel line could run smoothly but not develop full power. The human equivalent to this inefficiency, as an example, could be fatigue and shortness of breath when walking or climbing a flight of stairs.

Atherosclerosis is a slow, progressive narrowing of the coronary artery. When the lumen, the inside cavity of the vessel, has lost about 75 percent or more of its area, the lack of sufficient oxygenated blood to the heart muscle will result in angina (chest pain) during exertion. Women may experience very different symptoms, including neck pain, back pain, and fatigue.

But what happens with total artery obstruction? Just imagine a completely blocked fuel line or fuel filter at twenty thousand feet above ground level. Your engine stops, and the amount of damage will depend on where you are and how effectively emergency procedures are followed.

Why does a normal coronary artery become blocked?

A normal artery is a pliable, flexible structure made up of three layers:

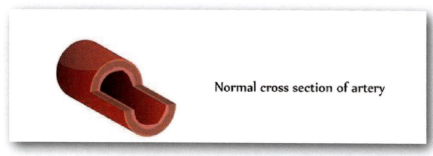

Normal cross section of artery

©Tefi/Shutterstock.com

The intima. A single layer of flat endothelial cells (the endothelium); a layer of collagen, proteoglycans, and glycoproteins; and a subendothelial space of loose connective tissue. This, the innermost layer or lining of the vessel, is where most of the action occurs in vascular disease.

The media. Composed of smooth muscle fibers and other connective tissue elements, these structures make up the wall of the vessel.

The adventitia. The outermost layer that holds the vasa vasorum (a network of vessels that supply blood to the artery itself) and nervi vasorum (autonomic nerve fibers that control arterial smooth muscle contraction).

Unlike the static fuel lines in your aircraft that accumulate debris on the surface of the interior, arterial narrowing is caused by the buildup of cholesterol and cellular material *under* the endothelial lining—in the intima—that then pushes up the endothelium and compresses the lumen of the artery.

The endothelium is not a static structure. It might, in fact, be considered an organ with multiple functions.[4] This single layer of cells is responsible for establishing a barrier that will allow passive diffusion of water and CO_2 and selective absorption of nutrients. Endothelial cells can make and secrete substances that prevent clotting in the normal vessel; modulate arterial dilation and constriction; and regulate cell growth, migration of white blood cells, and immune function. Endothelial cells have receptors (sites on the cell surface that accept a certain molecule) for cholesterol; insulin, which regulates blood sugar; and histamines, which respond to allergens, dilating vessels and making them leaky.[5]

Before going further, let's talk about cholesterol, the "C" word. Coronary artery disease does not happen without cholesterol. Is there really good and bad cholesterol? No. It's all about quantity and quality. What is cholesterol? Cholesterol is a steroid alcohol that is made by and utilized by every cell of your body for energy, cell-membrane maintenance, and steroid-hormone synthesis. Steroid hormones, by the way, include testosterone and estrogen. So, you see, cholesterol is critical for normal body function. Most of your cholesterol is produced by the liver or other cells—about 75 percent—whereas only about 25 percent comes from what you eat.[6] Eating eggs is bad? Fuggeddaboudit!

Cholesterol molecules are not water soluble and need to be transported throughout the body via carrier proteins, or apolipoproteins. There are multiple versions of these proteins. Apolipoproteins (ApoA and ApoB) are the carriers for HDL (high-density lipoproteins), VLDL (very low-density lipoproteins), LDL (low-density lipoproteins), IDL (intermediate-density lipoproteins), and Lp(a) (lipoprotein a).

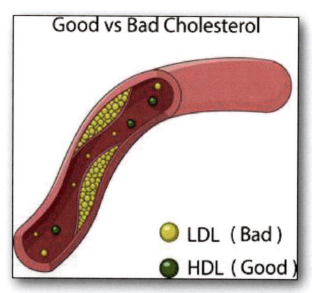
©Teguh Mujiono/Shutterstock.com

Cholesterol, specifically ApoB bearing LDL particles, is attached to the arterial endothelium and absorbed into the subendothelial space of the artery. It is suggested that ApoB absorption tends to occur at sites of endothelial injury, such as at artery branch points where shear, or unaligned, forces related to blood flow are at work. But the entire arterial tree is subject to pulsatile forces originating in the beating heart. Under normal conditions there is a balance between the mechanical forces of blood flow and the protective biochemical changes in the vessel lining, the endothelium. In a healthy individual, the endothelium adapts in response to mechanical pulsation stimulus, maintaining a pliable vessel. However, in situations when blood flow is low, which can happen due to inactivity, or when, oppositely, there are prolonged excessive shear forces, which occur in hypertensive individuals, the balance of forces is disrupted and results in changes in the vessel wall and lumen.[7, 8] To drive the point home further, think about a winding river. The water currents at the center of the river are different from the current near the banks, where flow is slower and eddy currents slowly remodel the riverbank as well as deposit debris. Similar forces are at work in your arteries where either abnormally high or low blood flow will affect the vulnerability of vessel wall, stimulating formation of plaque.

Fat entering the coronary artery wall triggers the endothelial cells to produce free radicals that oxidize the lipoproteins and secrete a substance that entices white blood cells (monocytes) to enter the intima and transform into macrophages, which are the body's disposal cells. Macrophages clean up debris, absorb the LDL particles, and enlarge, and these fat-distended cells are then called foam cells. This is the crossroads for development of heart disease. If the number of ApoB LDL particles is reduced, it is possible to recycle the fatty acids out of the subendothelial space. This is accomplished when apolipoprotein A (ApoA) bearing HDL recycles excess cholesterol back to the liver and gut. (This is why high HDL is a good thing.) If, however, the number of small, dense LDL particles is not reduced, the plaque continues to enlarge.[9, 10]

Size matters, but quantity matters more. Small LDL particles are absorbed through the endothelium in amounts almost two times greater than large LDL particles; however, with too many fat particles, the recycling process gets overwhelmed, and macrophages break down and start releasing toxic chemicals that promote necrosis. Necrosis occurs when cell death releases debris and toxic compounds, resulting in inflammation such as what might be seen in your skin after an injury. Your body's normal healing mechanisms will work to heal the lesion by forming a fibrous cap over the necrotic plaque. These lesions can calcify, allowing for identification on computerized axial tomography (CT) scan. Under circumstances that are not completely understood, the fibrous covering of some plaques, termed "vulnerable plaques," will thin and rupture. This releases substances in the blood-vessel lumen that inhibit the normal anticlotting mechanisms of the endothelial cells, resulting in formation of a blood clot that blocks the blood flow to the heart muscle and culminates in an acute event—a heart attack.

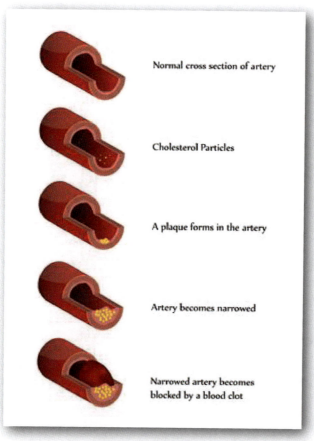

©Tefi/Shutterstock.com

Now, it sounds like this is a clear-cut process, but the fact is that it is intricately intertwined with functions of the liver, pancreas, adipose (fat), and skeletal tissue as well as maladapted mechanisms for containing inflammation. What I just described to you—the heart attack—is the end point of years of a combination of inappropriate food choices, lack of physical activity, inadequate sleep, chronic stress, smoking, and other environmental exposures that alter endothelial function. The operative word here is "inflammation." Type 2 diabetes, neurodegenerative diseases such as Alzheimer's disease, and many cancers all have roots in chronic low-level inflammation. So, if you can prevent or reverse chronic inflammation, can you avoid degenerative disease?

CHAPTER 3

Human Factors

> Tattaglia's a pimp. He never could've outfought Santino. But I didn't know until this day that it was Barzini all along.
> —VITO CORLEONE IN *THE GODFATHER*

It was not immediately obvious to Vito Corleone exactly which of the opposing mafiosi was his true enemy, but a little waiting and listening gave him the information. There are thousands of research studies investigating the cause, prevention, and treatment of coronary artery disease published over decades. So why is cardiovascular disease still the number-one killer worldwide? What increases the number of small LDL particles, and what is the trigger that initiates the deposition of fat into a blood vessel?

Unfortunately, there is not just one biological racketeer at the root of coronary artery disease. However, I can narrow it down to the two most important modifiable factors: *diet* and *exercise*. The interplay of what and how much you eat and how many hours a day you sit are at the top of a cascade of intertwined biological processes that control sugar and fat utilization and, if unbalanced, will lead to coronary artery disease. Genetics definitely comes into play here, and inherited traits are the cards you are dealt, but the expression of genes can be modified with diet and exercise. It was diet and exercise all along.

If you accept the theory that the human being evolved as a hunter-gatherer, it is easier to understand that our body systems are not designed to collapse in front of a TV set or sit immobile with only fingers moving on a computer keyboard. You can text on your smartphone all day long, but I can assure you that exerting the very small muscles in your hands does not offset the lack of using the large muscles of your hips and legs. All of our physiological processes were developed for metabolic flexibility to maintain stamina and survival in times of both famine and plenty. We have complex mechanisms for generation and storage of energy and can utilize proteins, fats, and carbohydrates as fuel. So unlike your airplane that will just spill fuel on the ground like the Exxon Valdez if overfilled, your body will make use of all nutrients that are loaded on in excess of what it actually needs. This means that nutrients will be stored and stored and stored—in your liver, abdomen, and muscles; around your heart; and both around and *in* your arteries.

The best way to understand this is by looking at a condition that is the direct result of low energy expenditure and high input of the wrong fuel: metabolic syndrome (MetS).

This topic could fill a book. The best definition I have found for the condition is given by Dr. Japinder Kaur in a review article published in 2014 in *Cardiovascular Research and Practice*: "Metabolic syndrome is defined by a constellation of interconnected physiologic, biochemical, clinical, and metabolic factors that directly increase the risk of cardiovascular disease, Type 2 diabetes mellitus, and all-cause mortality."[11] Get that? "All-cause mortality" is death from any cause! I'm sure you would agree that this is a condition to avoid.

Abdominal obesity, elevated serum triglycerides, low serum HDL, and elevated blood pressure are the hallmarks of metabolic syndrome. The National Cholesterol Education Program (NCEP/ATPIII) defines metabolic syndrome as the presence of three of the following five clinical findings:

1. Waist circumference of forty inches or larger in men and thirty-five inches or larger in women
2. Serum triglyceride level 150 mg/dl or greater
3. HDL cholesterol less than 40 mg/dl in men or less than 50 mg/dl in women; or drug treatment for low HDL
4. Blood pressure 130/85 or greater; or drug treatment for hypertension
5. Fasting blood glucose of 100 mg/dl or greater; or treatment for elevated fasting blood glucose

How does this happen? If you look at the following flowchart, you will see that a combination of factors working together lead to the metabolic consequences of too much of the wrong type of fuel. This is a problem with weight and balance.

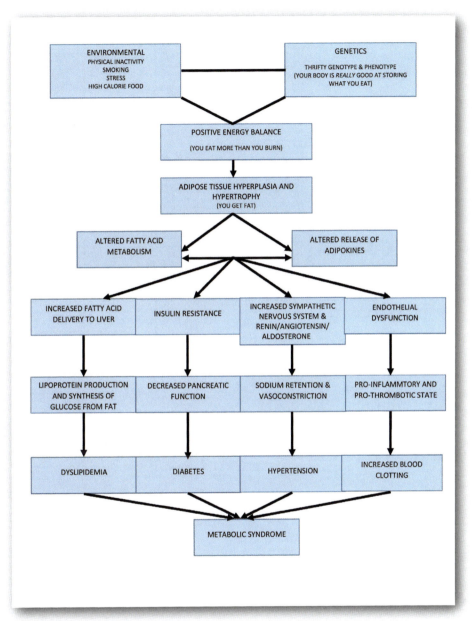

Metabolic Syndrome Flowchart: Adapted from Kaur, "A Comprehensive Review."[12]

Unless you loved biochemistry in school, stop at "Adipose tissue (fat cells) hyperplasia (increase number) and hypertrophy (increase size)." Here comes the Goodyear Blimp! And here's another good reason to take a hard look at this chart. Starting in March 2015, the Federal Aviation Administration, addressing industry concerns of the Congressional and National Transportation Safety Board, has included screening for obstructive sleep apnea as part of the pilot medical-certification exam. Obesity, defined as a BMI greater than thirty-five, is the number-one item on the list of factors associated with high risk for sleep apnea. So what is sleep apnea? According to the National Heart, Lung, and Blood Institute, the condition is marked by pauses in breathing or shallow breathing during sleep, resulting in disruption of the normal sleep pattern and excessive sleepiness during the day. Bad sleep leads to reduced reaction times, impaired judgment, and documented increase in accidents. Sleep apnea is also an independent risk factor for cardiovascular disease. (Read more about sleep apnea in chapter 5.)

Your BMI can be determined by using any of the available calculators or charts available on the Internet. Or if you are more inclined to do the math, use this:

BMI = (weight in pounds / (height in inches × height in inches)) × 703

One more piece of medical jargon you should be familiar with is "insulin resistance." This is one of the hallmarks of metabolic syndrome. Insulin is a hormone secreted by the pancreas, an organ that lies behind your stomach. The role of insulin is to control the glucose level in the blood. In response to rising blood-sugar (glucose) levels that occur after a meal, the pancreatic cells make and secrete the insulin hormone. Insulin increases glucose uptake in fat cells, muscle cells, and liver cells. The excess glucose (i.e., the amount ingested in excess of what your body needs to generate required energy) is stored in the liver and muscles as glycogen. With increased energy demands, the liver can break down the glycogen back into glucose.

I have simplified this process, but think about what this means. Your body has this elegant system to clear nutrients from the blood. Now let's put this in aviation terms. When you have an airplane properly trimmed, you are not fighting the controls, and everything is in balance, including your grip on the controls. The body, too, needs to be properly *trim* and healthy. There is a limit to the pancreas's capacity to keep up with overeating. The pancreas will increase insulin production, but at some point the demand exceeds output, and the result with be increased blood-sugar levels, increased liver glycogen (fat), increased fat in muscle, and increased fat deposits in your body as well as direct effects on the vascular endothelium.[13, 14] This is not just a problem in the United States. The International Diabetes Federation estimates that 20–25 percent of the world population has metabolic syndrome.[15] Metabolic syndrome not only increases the risk of heart disease but also increases the risk for development of type 2 diabetes.[16, 17, 18, 19] You must have seen the TV commercials of all the happy, overweight diabetic people taking whatever drug that decreased their glucose levels but also might have caused unwanted side effects. Would it not be easier to prevent the disease in the first place? Breaking the chain in the MetS flowchart above "POSITIVE ENERGY BALANCE" will prevent the ill effects of too much adipose tissue. So, just like controlled flight into terrain, metabolic syndrome is completely preventable.

Weight and Balance

What happens when we don't balance calorie intake with energy output?

As I researched this book, the question arose: If activity level is critical, what happens to people who can't walk? People who have suffered spinal cord injuries are at increased risk for cardiovascular disease. It was previously thought that higher rates of heart disease in spinal-injury patients was the result of better therapies for people suffering paralysis, resulting in increased life expectancy and, of course, cases of age-related heart disease. But this is not the case. Compared to the general population, paralyzed people show higher incidence of having low serum HDL (the good guys), high serum LDL (the bad guys), elevated triglycerides, abnormalities of glucose metabolism, and high blood pressure. The abnormal lipid profiles can occur even in a disabled person with a normal BMI, suggesting that the cause is not just increased body fat.[20, 21, 22, 23, 24, 25] With the loss of function of the largest muscle groups in the body—the abdominal, back, buttock, and leg muscles—diet and exercise become critical for maintenance of health in this group of people.

What about astronauts? Well, you say, why am I asking this question? Early Skylab experiments demonstrated astronauts' loss of bone density and lower-extremity muscle strength, as well as cardiovascular deconditioning, due to loss of gravitational loading.[26, 27] Our bodies have evolved to exist in the earth's 1 g gravitational field. In the absence of the earth's gravity, normal body processes go awry.[28] In order to study the effects of weightlessness, NASA developed experiments to mimic the environment in space. It was found that subjects placed on bed rest suffer the same physiologic effects that astronauts experience from weightlessness. Even young and healthy individuals if placed on bed rest will experience cardiovascular deconditioning and loss of bone density and muscle. The body builders reading this will know that skeletal muscle is made up of type 1 (slow-twitch) and type 2 (fast-twitch) fiber types. The slow fibers do the work of maintaining posture, and the fast fibers perform high-power rapid movements.[29] Without the stimulus of gravity, muscle cells will atrophy, and the postural slow fibers will convert to the fast-fiber type. Why is this bad? Slow-twitch muscle fibers are more resistant to fatigue and use fats for fuel. Fast-twitch fibers use glucose and do not have the capacity for sustained activity. This is great for short-term intense activity; however, for sustained activity, anaerobic fat metabolism is needed. Muscle atrophy and conversion of slow-type muscle fibers to fast-type fibers drastically changes metabolism as muscles lose the ability to use fat for energy. The metabolic effects of a lower proportion of slow-twitch muscle fibers include lower HDL (good) cholesterol and insulin resistance.[30, 31]

Bed-rest studies show that fat accumulates in the muscle even if food intake is less than the required intake for energy balance. This occurs as a result of the loss of the fat-utilizing slow-muscle fibers but is also possibly due to direct change of mesenchymal cells in the muscles into fat cells as a result of loss of gravitational stimulus.[32] What this means is that atrophied muscle cannot use fat effectively for metabolism. So where does the fat go? Imagine, then, what is happening to your muscles when most of the day is spent sitting at work, watching TV, or working in front of a computer screen. If your muscles are not using fat for fuel, the fat will take up residence in other organs, including your arteries. A sedentary lifestyle, specifically sitting for more than ten hours a day, has been identified as an independent risk factor for coronary heart disease. We are the beneficiaries and the victims of technology. Inactivity is as destructive to physiology as spending time in an orbiting space station.

In order to fully comprehend the downstream effects of sitting most of the day and consuming too much food, you need to understand that, with the exception of your fingernails and hair, every tissue of your body is biologically active (i.e., capable of secreting substances [hormones] into your bloodstream that act either locally or at other distant sites). Skeletal muscles and fat cells secrete biologically active compounds, so these tissues are also considered endocrine organs, just like your thyroid gland. What does this mean? Your fat cells are not passive depots of storage, and muscle cells; as we've just learned, they do more than produce great abs and thighs.

Adipose Tissue: Your Fat Cells in Action

There are fat cells beneath your skin that make up subcutaneous fat. Within your abdomen, between your organs, and in a structure called the "omentum"—a drape of fatty tissue that lies in the anterior abdomen covering your organs—there is visceral fat. It is known that subcutaneous fat cells (under the skin) are metabolically inert, whereas visceral fat (everywhere else) functions as an organ, growing vessels and releasing hormones (adipokines) into the bloodstream that directly promote the development of vascular disease.

So how does someone go from looking like a fighter jet to loking like a blimp?

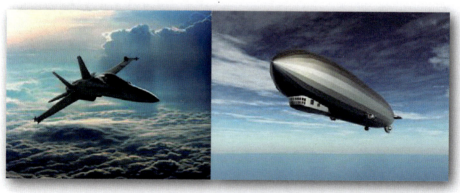

©Emilia Ungur/Shutterstock.com   ©Michael Rosskothen/Shutterstock.com

There is no magic here. Input of too much calorie-dense food (typically high-glycemic foods and excessive dietary fats), when not balanced by energy output through resistance and aerobic activity, results in increasing deposits of visceral fat.

What actually happens is that each fat cell enlarges to accept more fat, and with increasing volume, blood vessels are generated to maintain delivery of oxygen and nutrients. Blood supply may not keep up with the demand, resulting in an insufficient supply of oxygen to the fat tissue. This is hypoxia. Now, pilots are well aware of the neurological effects of hypoxia at high altitudes. Hypoxia at altitude is an insidious process. An individual may be totally unaware that his or her cognitive functions are being significantly reduced. Hypoxia in visceral fat is similarly lethal because the malfunction happening at the cellular level cannot be detected. Low oxygen stimulates the fat cells to secrete free fatty acids and hormones called adipokines. If you refer back to the metabolic syndrome flow chart, you will see that adipokines are bad actors. These inflammatory substances disrupt insulin sensitivity and energy metabolism and promote the progression of atherosclerosis.[33, 34, 35]

But there is at least one substance secreted by visceral fat that has positive effects. This is adiponectin. This hormone increases insulin sensitivity, lowers circulating free fatty acids, inhibits inflammatory molecules, and has a direct protective effect on blood vessels.[36, 37] Low adiponectin levels are present in type 2 (adult-onset) diabetics and are predictive of cardiovascular disease in patients with diabetes. It is possible to raise adiponectin levels by engaging in moderate- to high-intensity exercise training.[38, 39, 40, 41, 42]

Skeletal Muscle
Six-pack abs are doing more for you on the inside than on the outside.

A large amount of published data indicates that exercise is beneficial for people with metabolic syndrome, cancer, heart disease, arthritis, and just about any chronic condition you can name.

Skeletal muscle—the muscles attached to your bones—makes up the largest organ in the body. Contracting muscles use up nutrients and also produce and secrete myokines, hormone-like molecules that can communicate with other organs such as your liver and fat cells. Currently, seven of these compounds have been identified and are being studied.[43] One of these myokines is interleukin six (IL-6). Contracting muscles need nutrients for energy, and they produce IL-6, which acts in the muscle to increase fat metabolism and muscle-glucose uptake. IL-6 also stimulates the liver to make more glucose for muscle fuel, and it stimulates fat cells, breaking them down to produce more fuel for the contracting muscles. Compound this with what you have already learned about muscle atrophy and changes in how muscles process fuel, and you have begun to understand why the rate of heart disease remains high in our very sedentary society. Without contracting muscles, glucose and fats have no departure route. Moreover, insulin sensitivity is directly proportional to muscle (lean body) mass.[44] If you eat more than your muscles utilize, your body experiences a situation similar to the morning rush-hour traffic at any tunnel or bridge crossing when every approach and alternate route can be backed up for miles. So in an unexercised body, where do you think all the excess fuel ends up? It *backs up* in the liver, muscles, and abdomen, as well as around your heart and in your blood-vessel walls!

CHAPTER 4

Recommendations for Health

> Speed is life. Altitude is life insurance.
> —Old pilot adage

When things go awry, the more altitude you have, the more likely you will be able to either correct the problem or glide to an acceptable landing spot. Of course, this assumes you know what you are doing in the first place. Great pilots can feel the airplane and instinctively know how to manage an emergency. Take, for example, "Sully," Sullenberger's landing in the Hudson River. I don't think the outcome would have been the same if Sullenberger had been a low-time pilot and had done only the FAA-required minimum of three takeoffs and three landings in three months.

Great pilots fly often and are always in tune with what's going on both inside and outside the cockpit. This doesn't just happen. So does maintaining your health. There is no magic pill. There is no quick, easy fix. It takes time, repetition, and discipline.

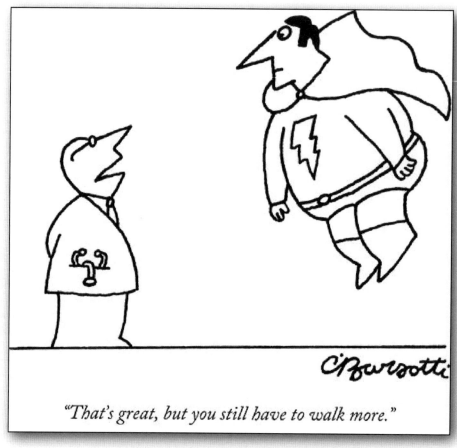

"That's great, but you still have to walk more."

©Charles Barsotti/The New Yorker Collection/The Cartoon Bank.

Exercise

I recently performed an aviation physical on a high-time corporate pilot who was bemoaning the fact that he was scheduled for an eighteen-hour trip in a Gulfstream 4. He explained that "back in the day" he and his copilot would take breaks and do a hundred push-ups. Youth and testosterone are wonderful things! And then he told me that his lady friend was complaining that now, when he was home between those long-haul flights, he preferred to do nothing. Fatigue? Sure, but perhaps this was a prelude to some problems downstream. Fortunately for him, his lady friend was keeping him motivated and off the couch. If you are working a five- or even seven-day week, or traveling in and out of different time zones, how do you fit exercise into your schedule? Health clubs may provide some motivation but can be expensive. Home gyms tend to collect dust.

Harold Reilly, a physiotherapist and proponent of drugless natural therapies whose clients included political, entertainment, and literary greats—including Nelson Rockefeller, Bob Hope, Marilyn Monroe, and Robert Frost—was once asked what the best exercises were. He responded, "The ones that you do." Pretty good advice. A better way to look at this is to consider what it takes to maintain proficiency in flying an airplane. For the general aviation pilot, the standard is three takeoffs and three landings within ninety days and in the type of aircraft usually flown. Commercial pilots are required by the FAA to undergo recurrent training in a simulator of the aircraft flown every six to twelve months, depending on the airline. For those of you who are nonpilots, you will be happy to know that this is a training requirement for the guys and gals in the cockpit to continue flying passengers. It requires a minimum two separate four-hour sessions to evaluate not only flight crew coordination and decision making but also to experience simulations of various emergencies, including engine loss at takeoff, approaches in limited visibility on takeoff, or landing in high winds. To maintain good health, recurrent training of the *body* is also needed—we need to train our muscles to support the rest of our bodies.

It is clear that physical activity can prevent vascular disease by improving lipid metabolism, preventing or reversing metabolic syndrome, and benefiting blood pressure.

The American Heart Association (AHA) recommends "at least thirty minutes of moderate-intensity aerobic activity at least five days a week or at least twenty-five minutes of vigorous aerobic activity at least three days per week or, a combination of moderate and vigorous activity with moderate to high-intensity muscle-strengthening activity at least two days per week for additional health benefits. To lower cholesterol and blood pressure, forty minutes of moderate- to vigorous-intensity aerobic activity three or four times a week." Moderate-intensity activity is defined as any activity similar to walking at three to four miles per hour.[45]

But what about the rest of the day? If, in fact, the remainder of your day is spent sitting, the thirty or forty minutes of any intensity exercise may blunt the physiologic effects of sitting but not enough to prevent heart disease. A study published in the journal *Metabolism* showed that just one day of sitting—even if food intake was reduced to match energy output—resulted in reduced insulin effect in young, healthy men and women.[46] Another study from Maastricht University Medical Center in the Netherlands evaluated the effects on insulin action and lipids in eighteen healthy, young adults divided into three separate activity groups.[47] One group sat for fourteen hours, the second group sat thirteen hours with one hour of vigorous exercise, and the third group sat eight hours but divided the other six hours into two hours of standing and four hours of walking. Remarkably, the last group did best in all categories. Moreover, it was determined that the one hour of vigorous exercise performed by the group 2 subjects did not compensate for the thirteen hours of sitting and its negative effects on lipids and insulin. Before you get too depressed, simply breaking up sessions of sitting with a short two-minute walk at two miles per hour every twenty minutes can substantially reduce the ill effects of prolonged sitting.[48]

Vascular disease prevention, then, can be as simple as taking walks during a workday. Avoiding a sedentary lifestyle and remaining active is key. But how do you know if you are active enough or too sedentary? As I was writing this book, sitting in front of my computer doing the exact thing I am preaching against, I decided to find out for myself.

I invested in a FitBit, a little device that tracks how many steps you take in a day and interacts with a website that graphically displays your activity. (I am not a paid spokesperson.) There are many alternative pedometers as well as cell-phone apps that can track number of steps. These devices can also monitor sleep and heart rate.

The commonly touted recommendation for optimal health is to take ten thousand steps a day; anything less than five thousand steps is considered low activity.[49] Ten thousand steps is about five miles of walking. This number, however is not based on any specific scientific research but was part of marketing of a pedometer that was developed in Japan in the 1960s. Thinking about this in another way, the number of steps taken in any given day equates to time not sitting. There is nothing so motivating as seeing exactly how active—or for that matter, inactive—you are in a given day. I was not happy to realize how little walking I did in a typical workday and have since made an effort to get up from my desk periodically and walk up to the top floor of the hospital.

Although the ten-thousand-step goal may not be absolute science, research has shown that people who consistently walk five thousand steps or less every day exhibit a variety of metabolic disturbances that are known to increase heart-disease risk. These include increased BMI, insulin resistance, and higher C-reactive protein (a blood-test marker of inflammation).[50, 51] The small monetary investment in a pedometer may pay for itself multiple times over if seriously used; it can provide incentive to get out of that chair! Choose simple, healthy actions like taking the stairs instead of the elevator, parking your car as far away from an entrance as possible, or, for you commercial or corporate pilots, rotating responsibility for the preflight walk-around. Walking is free, unlikely to cause injury, and possible anywhere.

Another solution to the ravages of sitting is simply standing up. Dr. Joan Vernikos, former director of NASA's Life Sciences Division, in her book *Sitting Kills, Moving Heals*, explains how gravity works synergistically with our body systems to keep us fit and healthy. She explains that standing up (i.e., rising against the 1 g force we live in) multiple times in the course of an hour is perceived by the body as multiple stimuli, whereas standing for a prolonged period is perceived as only one stimulus. Think of how children play—or at least how most played "back in the day" before electronic devices. Slow and rapid starts and stops, jumps, short sprints, and so on. Adults should keep this image in mind when they get up to move. When I was a kid, it was a summer Saturday ritual for my father to hand-wash the car. Think about all the total-body motion that is involved in that process. I still find this a very relaxing and almost meditative exercise. There is an advantage to approaching other chores with the mind-set that a job is not a burden but a form of exercise, with the added benefit that you get something done!

OK, so let's return to the American Heart Association recommendations. What do you gain from aerobic and weight-training exercises? Aerobic and endurance-type exercises will increase your slow-twitch muscle fibers. We know that's a good thing because it will directly improve insulin sensitivity and cholesterol levels.

What is moderate and vigorous exercise? The American College of Sport Medicine provides easily understandable guidelines:[52]

- Moderate-intensity aerobic endurance exercise increases your heart rate. A brisk walk will do this.
- Vigorous-intensity exercise, such as jogging, will increase heart rate and cause rapid breathing.

Those who frequent the gym and run on treadmills are familiar with the concept of maximal heart rate. Your maximal heart rate is 220 minus your age. The American Heart Association recommends targeting exercise heart rates between 50 and 85 percent of your maximal heart rate. There are many heart-rate calculators available on the Internet, and apps are available for smartphones. A few examples are included in the appendix.

There are specific benefits of both aerobic exercise and resistance or weight training. My opinion is that both types of activity should be heartily embraced. As we age, we lose muscle mass and tend to gain body fat. This is considered a normal part of aging, but perhaps it is also related to decreased activity. Resistance training will help maintain muscle mass. Remembering that insulin sensitivity is directly proportional to muscle mass, it seems a good idea to preserve the muscles you have. Resistance training can reduce resting blood pressure and have beneficial effects on blood lipids, raising HDL and lowering LDL cholesterol.[53, 54] An additional benefit of weight training is increased bone-mineral density, which helps maintain bone strength, an advantage for both women and men. And resistance training has been shown to generate distinct mental-health benefits, including reduction of fatigue, anxiety, and depression.[55, 56, 57] Aerobic exercise is effective in reducing excess visceral and liver fat and can also decrease insulin resistance. For overweight, sedentary people, a combination of both types of exercise has been shown to provide the most robust improvements in waist circumference, blood pressure, and serum triglycerides, the factors that indicate metabolic syndrome.[58]

Fuel: What and How Much to Eat

I love old books. Although quickly becoming extinct, there are a few "old book" bookstores that remain viable due to clientele who still like the feeling of turning pages and are looking for either a bargain or a treasure. I tend to migrate to the medical- and science-book sections in these shops to investigate how diagnosis and treatment has changed—or maybe how it hasn't changed—in the last one hundred years. I came across a book titled *Starving America*, written by Alfred W. McCann in 1912. It exposed the behind-the-scenes workings of the growing commercial-food industry in the United States.[59]

Surprisingly, some of what Mr. McCann described so long ago remains relevant today. In chapter 12, McCann explains that our diet should consist of "whole foods": a variety of whole-grain breads, vegetables, and fruits, rather than foods processed to enhance taste and shelf life. That was over one hundred years ago. Since then, the rates of obesity have skyrocketed, and the incidence of degenerative diseases, despite advances in medicine, has not declined. The fact is that in the United States, we are constantly barraged with advertisements for food. We eat too much and too often, and we have an overabundance of easily accessible processed and fast foods. To compound the problem, much data indicates that mineral content has been reduced in the soils in which we grow our food. The challenge of feeding the growing world population continues to be the impetus for innovations in industrial farming. It happens that industrial farming practices adopted in the United States and United Kingdom, designed to increase crop yield, result in reduction of minerals in some vegetables and fruits. The complex nature of soil chemistry, vegetation, and how our bodies process plant foods and nutrients is well beyond the context of this book. The bottom line is that the mineral content of many US-grown fruits and vegetables, as well as of crops all over the world, is less than it was fifty years ago.[60, 61, 62, 63, 64] With that in mind, a multivitamin and mineral supplement might be a good idea.

My paternal grandfather, nicknamed "CB," would start preparing the soil for his tomato garden in the fall. He dug into the earth two feet and then filled the area with fallen maple leaves and decayed material from the compost pile he kept at the edge of the property; he would thoroughly mix the soil with the died-off stalks of that year's tomato plants. He did this well into his eighties. Nothing tasted as marvelous as one of those fresh-picked tomatoes. How many times have you ordered a salad at a restaurant and been served a pale, tasteless tomato? Why does any of this matter? Our bodies need specific elements—vitamins, minerals, proteins, fats, and carbohydrates—for normal physiological functioning. These are provided by the soil—the plants that grow under the sun in the soil and the animals and marine life that consume the vegetation. Severe deficiency in any of these elements will ultimately result in diseases, such as rickets from vitamin D deficiency or scurvy from lack of vitamin C. But what about mild or borderline deficiency, or, for that matter, what about excess? Refer back to metabolic syndrome and the mechanisms of arterial plaque development. Although *overeating* is common in this country as a social event, an emotional outlet, or even a response to boredom, the reality is that eating is a requisite for health, and what you put in your mouth will determine how healthy you are.

Enough soapbox talk. How and what do you eat to prevent heart disease and other degenerative diseases? Think about what your grandparents, or even *their* grandparents, ate—and more importantly, what they didn't eat. The closest thing they had to a vending machine was the "automat" at Horn and Hardart in New York City and Philadelphia. This was a marvel restaurant where the behind-the-scenes kitchen staff filled a wall-sized, coin-operated vending machine with low-cost feshly made foods.

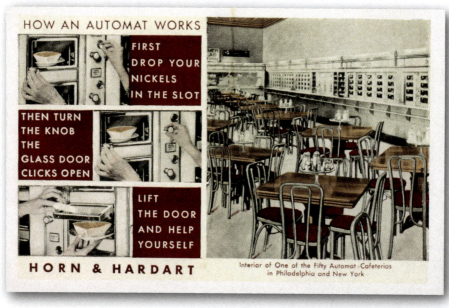

©Corbis Images

These were not the processed, plastic-packaged foods that fill our vending machines today. I remember being taken to the last still-operating shop in New York City and relishing the delicious piece of apple pie that I removed from the refrigerated stainless-steel cubicle after depositing a few quarters.

CB loved to tell stories about his boyhood in Italy and his mother's mill, which ground the local grain between huge discs of granite. He would refer in his Italian accent to "that goddamn stew-born donkey," which carried sacks of freshly milled grain and would frequently stop walking. On one of these occasions, my grandfather, in frustration, actually lit a fire under the donkey's belly to get him moving again. Not approved by the ASPCA, but at the time it ended up being too effective. The donkey ran off with the grain *and* my grandfather's little brother, who happened to be riding the donkey that day, holding on for dear life!

For centuries, whole grains, fresh vegetables, and olive oil, along with nuts and legumes, were the staples of the Italian peasant diet. And it turns out that this economical way of eating was the rule in the other countries bordering the Mediterranean Sea. After World War II, a landmark scientific study called "The Seven Countries Study"—which included Italy, the Greek Islands, Yugoslavia, the Netherlands, Finland, Japan, and the United States—was launched to investigate why the rates of heart disease were significantly lower in the Mediterranean region than in the then-prosperous United States. Through that study, published in 1953, Ancel Keys and the other researchers established the link between ingested cholesterol from butter, eggs, and red meat and the incidence of cardiovascular disease.[65, 66] There have since been many criticisms made concerning the structure of this study, including the deliberate exclusion of data from Switzerland, France, Sweden, and West Germany, where diets were high in saturated fats but the incidence of heart disease was low.[67] Brie and wine, anyone? It is my own opinion that other important factors, including walking hills and performing manual work, differentiated these European peoples from the postwar United States, where car travel and household conveniences, among other things, increased leisure time.

The components of a Mediterranean-style diet are depicted in the image below. There are many published food-pyramid graphics, but I prefer the Fundacion Dieta Mediterranea version presented on the next page.

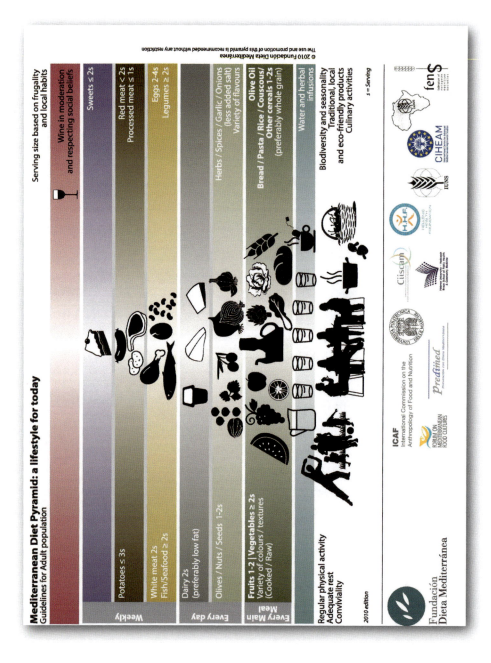

The recommendations suggest what should be consumed on a weekly basis, including a variety of vegetables, fruits, and whole grains daily. Olive oil is recommended as the principal source of dietary fat due to its nutritional content. Daily intake of about eight glasses of water, tea, or broth a day are suggested to maintain optimal hydration. Fish, white meat, eggs, and legumes provide a weekly source of protein. The typical Mediterranean diet does not use meat as the main meal ingredient and includes limited amounts of red and processed meats, but wine and sweets are included, making this guideline less onerous to adapt. What is particularly interesting, and I believe critical to the success of any lifestyle program, is the base of this pyramid, which includes activity, rest, conviviality, and seasonality of foods. In the upper right-hand corner is a definition of serving size that is based on "frugality and local habits." If you grew up in an Italian American family, as I did, one serving at the dinner table could probably have fed three people, so I think more emphasis should be given to the concept of frugality.

There are multiple websites, including the American Heart Association site, that define serving size of various foods. You will find that one serving is often much less than you might think. For example, one serving of grains is one slice of bread or one-half cup of cooked cereal—not a hoagie roll made with devitalized white flour, not a processed, sweetened boxed cereal that should be stocked in the dessert aisle of the supermarket. The USDA publishes a "choose my plate" graphic (http://www.choosemyplate.gov) that can help individuals visualize relative serving amounts of proteins, vegetables, grains, fruits, and dairy.

Although it should not be surprising that eating whole grains, fresh vegetables, fruits, and lesser amounts of protein is a healthy diet, medical researchers approach topics just like this one as an opportunity to investigate, publish, and prove or disprove the concept. Consequently, there have been a number of studies documenting the beneficial health effects of a Mediterranean-style diet. One such study is PREDIMED (PREvencion con Dieta MEDiterranea).[68] This six yearlong study included 7,447 people with no prior documented heart disease history but with significant cardiac risk factors such as type 2 diabetes, hypertension, elevated LDL cholesterol, low HDL cholesterol, obesity, or a family history of premature heart disease.

Study participants were split into three groups and placed on different diets: a Mediterranean diet with extra virgin olive oil (at least four tablespoons per day), a Mediterranean diet with nuts (at least three servings a day of walnuts, almonds, or hazelnuts), and a low-fat control-group diet. Interestingly, no physical activity recommendations were made. Both Mediterranean-diet groups showed a 30 percent reduction in risk for heart attack, stroke, and cardiovascular mortality in comparison to the control group. The diet group with extra virgin olive oil also had a slight reduction in overall mortality in comparison to the other two diet groups. Further study of these patient groups also showed reduction in onset of type 2 diabetes, decreased blood pressure, and improved lipid profiles. Significantly, reduction in arterial intimal thickening, delayed progression of arterial plaque, and actual regression of arterial plaque was documented in the Mediterranean diet groups. After following either Mediterranean diet for one year, participants displayed reduced serum markers of inflammation that are associated with arterial plaque formation and plaque instability.

Easier said than done? What do you eat when you are away from home for a twenty-eight-day stretch, you check in to some hotel at midnight, and you haven't eaten since the last time zone?

My suggestion is to plan ahead. Almonds and walnuts can be easily stored in a flight bag. Fresh and dried fruits are healthier options than pretzels and chips. Opt for water or tea instead of soda. Read labels, and stay away from high-fructose corn syrup, partially hydrogenated vegetables oils, and any ingredient you can't pronounce. If your only option is a cheeseburger, try to balance it with a salad, and skip the shake. Stay hydrated. The Mediterranean-diet pyramid recommends eight glasses of water or a near-equivalent every day. Adequate water is needed for the body's normal physiological processes. I have tried the sixty-four-fluid-ounce trial during a typical eight-hour workday, and the result was multiple trips to the bathroom. I was recently asked by one of my pilots if the eight-glass rule is true. My own opinion, not backed up by any science, is that it depends on your age, health status, environment, and activity level.

I have read innumerable articles about drinking water for skin health. But more important than the way you look is the way you think. Some evidence suggests that mild dehydration might negatively impact cognitive functioning.[69, 70, 71, 72] Mild dehydration is defined as about one to three pounds of fluid body weight loss. This is unlikely to happen in the cockpit but can occur with more vigorous daily activity. Thirst is the trigger to drink water, but I find that when I am focusing on work, as any pilot would be in the cockpit, it is easy to suppress or ignore this stimulus. Keep in mind that the liquid portion of your blood, plasma, is approximately 90 percent water, and plasma makes up about 50 percent of your blood volume. My suggestion is to try to consume the suggested eight glasses of water a day, keeping in mind that some foods will contribute to this volume. If your urine is dark amber, you are probably not hydrated enough. The United States Army

Health Command issues the following urine color chart to illustrate the variations in urine color with hydration as well as a fluid-replacement guide for recommendations of fluid intake per hour according to ambient temperature and workload.

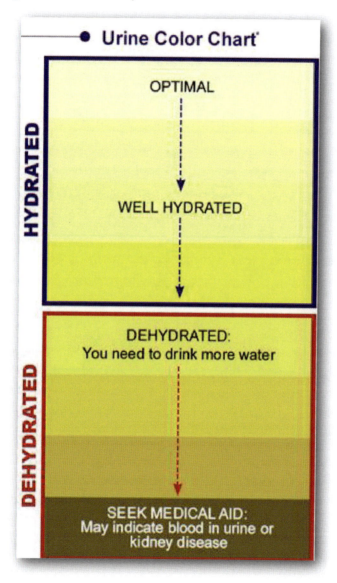

Fluid Replacement Guide

Heat Category	WBGT Index, (°F)	Easy Work Walking on hard surface, 2.5 mph, <30 lb. load; weapon maintenance, marksmanship training. Fluid Intake (quarts/hour)	Moderate Work Patrolling, walking in sand, 2.5 mph, no load; calisthenics. Fluid Intake (quarts/hour)	Hard Work Walking in sand, 2.5 mph, with load; field assaults. Fluid Intake (quarts/hour)
1	78° - 81.9°	½	¾	¾ (1)*
2	82° - 84.9°	½	¾ (1)*	1 (1¼)*
3	85° - 87.9°	¾	¾ (1)*	1 (1¼)*
4	88° - 89.9°	¾	¾ (1¼)*	1 (1¼)*
5	> 90°	1	1 (1¼)*	1 (1½)*

*Use the amounts in parentheses for continuous work when rest breaks are not possible. Leaders should ensure several hours of rest and rehydration time after continuous work. This guidance will sustain performance and hydration for at least 4 hours of work in the specified heat category. Fluid needs can vary based on individual differences (± ¼ qt/hr) and exposure to full sun or full shade (± ¼ qt/hr). Rest means minimal physical activity (sitting or standing) in the shade if possible. Body armor - add 5°F to WBGT index in humid climates. NBC (MOPP 4) - Add 10°F (Easy Work) or 20°F (Moderate or Hard Work) to WBGT Index. **CAUTION:** Hourly fluid intake should not exceed 1½ qts. Daily fluid intake should not exceed 12 qts.

I suspect that by now I have made Mediterranean diet converts of at least some of you. The Mediterranean countries are populated by peoples whose religions include ritual fasting. This is not merely a mode of self-sacrifice; it is actually beneficial to your health. Let's go back to the mechanisms of atherosclerosis. What is driving the small LDL particles? Excess glucose loads and storage of glycogen in liver and muscles drive development of metabolic syndrome, contributing to a microenvironment favorable for atherosclerosis development. Studies of people during and after fasting show that liver and skeletal-muscle glycogen decreases, insulin resistance reverses, and output of fatty acid from the liver is reduced. Fasting has beneficial effects on endothelial function, BMI, blood pressure, and lipid profiles, as well as arterial intimal thickness.[73, 74, 75] A recent research study placed nineteen healthy men and women on a plant-based, calorie-restricted diet that mimicked fasting for five consecutive days a month for three months; subjects exhibited reduced risk factors and markers of aging, diabetes, cardiovascular disease, and cancer.[76] Five days of strict, reduced food intake might be a bit of a challenge for most individuals. But the benefits of intermittent fasting can actually be achieved by eating six hundred calories per day (if male) or five hundred per day (if female) for two out of seven days.[77, 78] Yes, boys and girls, in the United States we eat too much and too often.

What if you know you have coronary artery disease? Is it possible to implement lifestyle changes that will actually result in regression of coronary artery plaque? It may be surprising to some of you, but the answer is yes. Dr. Dean Ornish, www.ornishspectrum.com, after almost forty years of research and study, has developed a comprehensive program, involving lifestyle and dietary changes, that has demonstrated published, positive results in patients with diagnosed coronary artery disease.[79, 80, 81] Adherents to this program experienced improvements in lipid profiles and actual documented decreases in the narrowing of diseased coronary arteries. This is a "boot camp," a long-term program that prescribes a strict low-fat, plant-based diet; aerobic exercise; strength training; stress management; and group support. The positive effects of this lifestyle program have been so well documented that the Centers for Medicare and Medicaid Services have granted Medicare reimbursement for the program. Since you now have an understanding of the drivers of heart disease, it should not be surprising that a program of this type would work. Like learning to fly, it requires time, commitment, and dedication.

An Apple a Day Keeps the Doctor Away

It might surprise (or maybe disgust) you to know that there are more microorganisms living on and in you than there are cells in your body. I am sure you have seen the TV commercials recommending probiotics or yogurt with "live cultures" for intestinal health. These products deliver live bacteria that will take up residence in your intestinal tract. Hundreds of different bacteria live in your intestines. The specific types depend on many factors, including genetics, mode of birth (babies delivered via C-section have different bacterial colonies than those born naturally), and medications, particularly antibiotics. More importantly, what you eat can change the proportion and composition of gut bacteria types, and the degree of diversity of your particular microbe colonies has significant repercussions on your overall health. The gut flora of a vegetarian is quite different from that of someone whose dietary mainstay is red meat. Intestinal bacteria, or microbiota, do more than just keep your digestive system "regular." Microbiota have a symbiotic relationship with you. You feed them; they digest fiber and complex carbohydrates, extract nutrients, and synthesize vitamins B12 and K and other metabolites. They are also involved in bile-acid metabolism and function to maintain the health of your intestinal lining, which creates a barrier against pathogenic (bad) bacteria.

There is increasing evidence that disruption in the proportions of certain types of intestinal bacteria can lead to obesity, type 2 diabetes, and cardiovascular disease as bacterial metabolites are produced and absorbed promoting insulin insensitivity and inflammation. The food you consume provides you with not only nourishment but also your microbiome. You are, in fact, eating for a few trillion. It is difficult to avoid getting too scientific on this topic, but simply put, overgrowth of specific bacteria in people who regularly consume red meat, for example, results in production of a molecule called TMAO (trimethylamine N-oxide), which is a major risk factor for atherosclerosis. There continues to be investigation on this topic, but it is clear that certain foods, particularly vegetables and fruits, have a beneficial effect on cholesterol and glucose metabolism. For example, apples are rich in insoluble fiber, pectin, and polyphenols. Some animal studies and one minor human study revealed that ingesting apples has a positive impact on gut bacteria, promoting decreased pathogenic strains and increased beneficial strains. Fiber represents the major energy source for microbiota. Beans, whole grains, fruits, and vegetables are the best sources of food for your microbiota. Considering the beneficial effects of a Mediterranean diet, which stresses intake of vegetables and fruit, it is likely that some, if not all, of the health-promoting diet results may actually be secondary to the actions of the gut bacteria. For a more complete discussion of this topic read *The Good Gut*, by Justin and Erica Sonnenburg, listed in Recommendations at the end of this book.

Stress

An important component of the Ornish program includes stress management.[82] Chronic mental stress is a driver of coronary artery disease. I have witnessed this in my own family.

My paternal grandfather, CB, lived to age ninety-two. He was still climbing on his roof and planting his garden until he ultimately died of what was assumed to be a heart attack while starting his lawn mower. My maternal grandfather, Poppa, died at the age of seventy-three of a ruptured aortic aneurysm. Both were born in Italy. Both avoided sweets and processed foods. Both were surrounded by their families. They came from two different families from different regions in Italy; they possessed differing genetic makeups and, more importantly, very different occupations.

CB made his living as a barber. He loved his work; in fact, after he had sold his business, at the age of eighty-six, he acquired a part-time job by telling the owner of the new establishment that he was only seventy-five years old. His shop was close to Brooklyn College in New York City, and his clients were professors and other neighborhood locals.

Poppa was CEO of a construction company. Builder of schools and hospitals in the boroughs of New York, friend and confidant of the New York power circle, he loved his work, ate healthy, and avoided desserts unless it was a birthday celebration. I remember, as a kid, walking across the street to my grandparents' house in the evening. Poppa always had an apple or pear after dinner. He peeled the fruit with a small knife and placed the spiral of the skin, intact, on his plate. I still can't do this. "Here, Jackie, eat this," he would say, handing me a beautifully sliced piece of apple or pear. I ate it because he was so pleased to share this beautiful ripe fruit with me. But I must admit: at the time I would have been happier with an

JACQUELINE BRUNETTI, MD

Oreo. The stress of a changing economy in the 1970s took its toll on the construction industry and Poppa.

What is the impact of emotional stress on your body? Whether at the controls or in a passenger seat, I am always fascinated by how the world looks at altitude. Think, for instance, how you feel in your automobile, in bumper-to-bumper traffic, when the radio traffic report gives you no indication of why you are traveling at five miles per hour rather than sixty-five. Or how do you feel when those lighted highway signs alert you that there is traffic at some exit several miles ahead? Frankly, I would prefer not to know and to have a few more moments of ignorant bliss. On the other hand, the traffic-helicopter pilot, at three thousand feet AGL, has quite a different vantage point. If we could understand health and disease from a thirty-thousand-foot perspective, I believe we would transform methods of fighting disease into programs for disease *prevention* and health maintenance.

I recently had the opportunity to spend an hour in a Falcon 700X simulator. For those of you who are not commercial pilots, this training simulator is a multi-million-dollar apparatus that reproduces the cockpit environment and the experience of flying—so convincingly that no matter how rational you think you are, you enter a realm of suspended disbelief. Like the movie *The Matrix*, the generated reality is your reality. I was extremely pleased with myself when I successfully "landed" the aircraft at the simulated JFK International Airport. If, however, I had been hooked up to a heart monitor, I know my heart and breathing rates would have read well above my baseline normal values. But, although I was exhilarated, the higher-time pilot in the right seat of the simulator explained he was actually anxious because he was not controlling the aircraft. Lack of control in any situation results in high stress levels.

I was fortunate to attend a lecture by Dr. Peter Hancock, Professor and Chair of the Department of Psychology, University of Central Florida, entitled "Who Will Fly in the Future: The Human Role in Automated Flight Spaces."

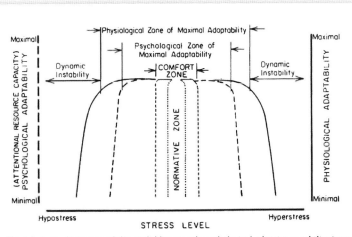

Figure 2. *Physiological adaptive capability (solid lines) and psychological adaptive capability (outer dashed lines: equated with attentional resource capacity) as functions of stress level. Embedded in these zones is a region of comfort sought by the active operator. A central normative zone describes a region in which compensatory action is minimized, as environmental input is insufficient to demand appreciable dynamic response. Within zones of maximal adaptability, negative feedback predominates. Outside stable limits, positive feedback induces dynamic instability that proceeds toward the breakdown of adaptive response and eventually functional failure.*

Courtesy of Hancock, "A Dynamic Model."[83]

Dr. Hancock explained how both high and low workloads can have ill effects on attention and ability. His graphic very clearly demonstrates that low-stress and high-stress situations are equally bad for performance.[84] I know that if I have a particularly slow day at work, I am actually annoyed if someone asks me to do something. The less you do, the less you want to do. This can be a problem in the cockpit, where all controls are automated and human input becomes infrequent. Constant vigilance is required to "stay ahead of the airplane." On the right side of Dr. Hancock's graph, we see that information overload and multitasking will equally result in instability, lack of control, and increased likelihood of error. We view automation as progress, a way to streamline processes and improve efficiency. Dr. Hancock's view is this: "If you build systems where pilots are rarely required to respond, when required, they will rarely respond." I happen to agree with this opinion. So what does this have to do with stress and heart disease?

We take for granted certain responses to external stimuli. I would bet that not one human being could ride a roller coaster without any changes in heart rate, breathing, or muscle tension. These are normal responses to fear that prepare your body for "fight or flight." In the case of the roller-coaster ride, this is welcomed and voluntary. Stress events, both psychological and somatic (bodily), are processed in the brain. Reflex stimulation of the autonomic nervous system and the hypothalamic-pituitary axis (HPA) result in increased heart rate, elevated blood pressure, and energy mobilization, as well as a release of cortisol that promotes mobilization of stored energy. You are then ready to "fight or run like heck."[85]

Mental or psychological stress produces both physiological and behavioral changes that are protective in an acute event but that can become damaging to your body if unchecked. As evidenced in the graphic below, chronic mental stress triggers mechanisms that lead to physiological changes that promote the development of heart disease.[86] If you refer back to the metabolic syndrome chart in chapter 4, you will see that chronic mental stress is as damaging to your body as too much food and too little activity. Approximately one-third of cases of acute myocardial infarction can be attributed to reactions to major life events, lack of control over life, financial issues, or other stress at work or home.[87]

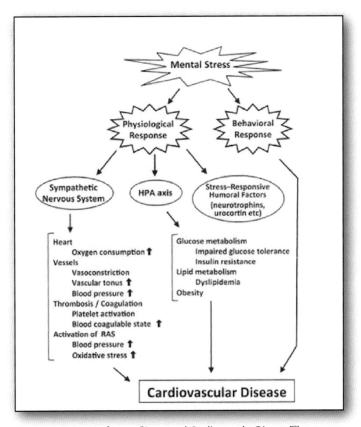

Courtesy of Inoue, "Stress and Cardiovascular Disease."[88]

Everyone can admit to some level of stress in daily life. It is lack of control over the stressor that contributes to the development of disease. More importantly, it is your interpretation of troubling or emotionally charged events that continues to drive the stress response. This is the cornerstone of mind-body medicine. Much of what occurs during the stress response is happening in primitive lower-brain structures and reflex loops in your spinal column. This can be modulated and overridden, however, by the higher-evolved cerebral cortical gray matter that is the center of thought and intention.

This is why meditation works. I must admit that every time I mention the word "meditation" to one of my pilots, I get blank looks, probably accompanied by the thought "She's really lost it now." But meditation need not be a cross-legged, lotus-position, becoming-one-with-the-universe experience. Meditation can be prayer, attention to breathing, a trip to the ocean, or anything that can interrupt the thoughts that generate toxic stress responses. Remember my telling you about washing the car in chapter 4? Any activity, chore or hobby that will divert your attention from perceived problem at hand can be a meditative experience. Always keep in mind that the culprit may not be reality but rather your *interpretation* of reality.

If meditation is not your cup of tea, you will be happy to know that exercise training, both aerobic and resistance, can blunt the effects of stress. Aerobic training will lower sympathetic nervous-system reactivity to stress, and both aerobic and resistance exercise have been shown to reduce inflammatory cytokine levels following exposure to mental stress.[89] If you think about it, this is another way to divert your attention but, more importantly, another incentive to get off the couch!

CHAPTER 5

Hazard Avoidance

Smoking

Don't start if you never did, and stop if you currently do. That's all. It is well known that nicotine is addictive. Cigarette smoke contains at least fifty carcinogens (compounds that cause cancer) and many other compounds that disrupt vasomotor activity, or the normal functioning of blood vessels; cause vascular dysfunction by direct effect on endothelial cells; promote oxidation of lipids; spur arterial plaque development; and enhance clotting. Remember the mechanisms in chapter 3? Cigarette smoke destroys lung tissue and increases the risk of lung, pancreatic, and urinary-tract cancers. Interestingly, smoking is more likely to affect the abdominal aorta and the arteries in your legs than the coronary arteries. And guess what? The arteries to the penis come from the branches of the aorta. And smoking also has a direct aging effect on skin. So if you don't care about your heart, maybe ED or facial wrinkles will be a *potent* inhibitor. Need I say more?

Partially Hydrogenated Vegetable Oil (Trans Fats)
Mayor Mike Bloomberg had the guts to ban trans fats in New York City restaurants in 2006. Far from being a power grab, this was a

significant step toward improving the health of New Yorkers by eliminating a substance that has been clearly evidenced to promote heart disease. The data was so compelling that the FDA followed suit; in November 2013, they issued this Federal Register notice: "Based on new scientific evidence and the findings of expert scientific panels, the Food and Drug Administration (FDA) has tentatively determined that partially hydrogenated oils (PHOs), which are the primary dietary source of industrially produced *trans* fatty acids, or *trans* fat, are not generally recognized as safe (GRAS) for any use in food based on current scientific evidence establishing the health risks associated with the consumption of *trans* fat, and therefore that PHOs are food additives." The decision to completely ban trans fats was finally been made in 2015; however, full compliance is not required by the FDA until 2018.

Trans fats are made commercially by heating liquid vegetable oils with metal catalysts and hydrogen to form shortening and margarine.[90] The resulting product is solid at room temperature and increases the shelf life of food products; it also allows food products to be manufactured less expensively. In an effort to satisfy consumer desires to reduce saturated fats, food manufacturers and restaurants replaced lard and tallow with trans-fat products. When I was about eight years old, my family was invited for breakfast at the summer home of a cardiologist friend. Remember: it was in the 1950s that the war on saturated fat began. I was thrilled to see a plate of pancakes placed in front on me. I enthusiastically spread what I thought was butter on these perfectly stacked pancakes, only to be horrified by the taste of margarine. When I protested, I was sternly told, "It's good for you!" Well, it definitely is not. With the push by the medical community to lower saturated fat, we all became victims of improvement!

There has been a building body of evidence since the 1970s that ingestion of trans fats is directly related to development of heart disease. Keep in mind that human physiology did not evolve to be able to process industrially molecularly altered fat. In pregnant women, trans fats cross the placenta and are excreted in breast milk. Trans fats compete with natural fatty acids in normal enzymatic reactions that produce prostaglandins and accumulate, with the exception of the brain, in body tissues.[91, 92, 93, 94] Prostaglandins are lipid compounds that have a variety of functions in the body, including constricting or relaxing the smooth muscles of arteries and adjusting platelet function to either promote or inhibit clotting; they also help regulate hormones and inflammation. Consumption of trans fats is associated with an increased risk of heart attack due, at least in part, to direct effects on lipids, as triglycerides and LDL cholesterol increase, while HDL cholesterol is reduced.[95, 96, 97, 98, 99]

Since 1999 the FDA has required food manufacturers to list the trans-fat content of food. Many manufactures have removed trans fats from their products and proudly state on their packaging, "no trans fats." But until there is full implementation of the FDA ban in 2018, the stuff is still out there. The Center for Disease Control website lists fried foods, snacks (microwave popcorn, etc.), frozen pies and pizzas, baked goods, margarines and spreads, ready-to use frosting, and coffee creamers as typical sources of trans fats. *Always read labels!*

High-Fructose Corn Syrup

High-fructose corn syrup (HFCS) is pervasive in the American diet. Fructose is a sugar that is cheaper than cane sugar and much sweeter.

Fructose occurs naturally in fruit, where is it bound chemically to glucose. HFCS used in commercial baking gives bread the appealing brown crust. Read the labels of carbonated beverages, ketchup, candy, jelly, packaged baked goods, canned fruits, and some dairy products—you *will* find high-fructose corn syrup. Unlike molasses, unprocessed brown sugar, or honey, HFCS, as well as processed white cane sugar, has no nutritional benefit. When you eat HFCS, you are getting a sugar load and calories without useful nutrients—unlike when you eat a piece of fruit, which provides fiber, vitamins, and minerals in addition to natural sugar. But it's not one glass of soda that will kill you; it is the cumulative effects of overloading your metabolism.

Fructose is handled differently by your body than glucose, which is the simplest sugar and acts as the building block of complex carbohydrates. Glucose is the fuel for energy in the body. It can be manufactured from breakdown of complex carbohydrates, and liver cells can produce it on demand. Fructose is metabolized in your body like alcohol. The chemical reactions are too complex to list here, but the end results are increased triglycerides, small LDL particles, and fat in liver cells; hepatic cell and muscle cell insulin resistance; and hypertension.[100, 101] This is the road to metabolic syndrome and obesity, both risk factors for heart disease.

Sugar also exerts a more direct effect on your body. Sugars react with proteins in your body to produce advanced glycation end products (AGE), and it has been demonstrated that fructose is actually more highly reactive than glucose.[102] These AGE compounds accumulate on DNA and collagen and are implicated in vascular, renal, and eye complications of diabetes as well as in the development of atherosclerosis.[103, 104, 105, 106] So this should be enough incentive to reduce your intake of sugar—and particularly high-fructose corn syrup. But, of course, this is easier said than done. If you are old enough to remember Walt Disney's animated film *Pinocchio*, you may recall Pinocchio's trip with Lampwick to Pleasure Island, a place where you can eat, drink, and do whatever strikes your fancy, all with ultimately bad consequences. Consuming sugar-laden foods and drinks is like a trip to Pleasure Island. Sugar directly acts on the pleasure centers of the brain, altering dopamine and opioid neurotransmission and increasing appetite.[107] The combination of sugar and fat is almost irresistible.

All this is not just theory. The regular consumption of sweetened beverages is associated with an increase in heart-disease risk due to adverse changes in lipid profiles, increased inflammatory markers, and decreased leptin.[108, 109, 110, 111] Remember that inflammation is a culprit of atherosclerosis development, and low leptin levels trigger excessive hunger. Perhaps New York's Mayor Mike Bloomberg was right on in his effort to limit the size of sweetened soft drinks to sixteen ounces with the Portion Cap Rule, a regulation that was overturned by the courts as unconstitutional.

Hypertension

High blood pressure, or hypertension, is a known risk factor for heart disease, stroke, and kidney failure. You will remember from chapter 3 that arteries are pliable but that under conditions of increased shear stress, the arterial wall will undergo remodeling. This is what happens with prolonged elevated blood pressure. Chronic exposure to elevated blood pressure will case the heart muscle to hypertrophy, just like your biceps following weight training.

A normal blood pressure (BP) is a reading of 120/80 or less. The upper number is the systolic pressure, or pressure when the heart contracts (systole), and the lower number is the diastolic pressure, reflecting the pressure in the arteries when the heart muscle relaxes (diastole). New medical guidelines for treatment of hypertension were set in 2014. For those aged sixty or older, a blood pressure of greater than or equal to 150/90 should be treated with appropriate blood-pressure-lowering drugs. Individuals under sixty years of age should seek treatment with blood pressures at or more than 140/90.[112]

A few commercial pilots who come to me for aviation medical examination get so anxious on the day of their scheduled exams that their initial blood-pressure readings and pulse are always high. After we talk for a while, I might coach the pilot to perform relaxation breathing exercises; I will retake the blood pressure a few times, and readings will decrease to the level acceptable to the FAA. I recommend to these pilots that they purchase a blood-pressure wrist cuff and record readings at home, and some even document by cell-phone photographs. These pilots have classic "white coat" hypertension, or elevated blood pressure in the clinic environment with normal readings at home.[113, 114] The condition perfectly demonstrates the adverse effects of anxiety. These pilots' fears of failing the test and losing their livelihood drive the stress response that you read about in chapter 5. The key to my job is to ensure that there is not any underlying *true* hypertensive disorder, and typically, I will recommend that an airman follow up with his or her private physician for further management. This is the FAA recommendation for blood-pressure readings above the FAA medical standard of 155/95. Treated hypertension is no reason for denial of medical certification, and if discovered on an aviation medical exam, the FAA has a simple pathway for certification after the airman initiates antihypertension medication; certification is possible just two weeks following initiation of therapy, as long as the airman shows no drug side effects and blood pressure is controlled and stable.

Vitamin D Deficiency

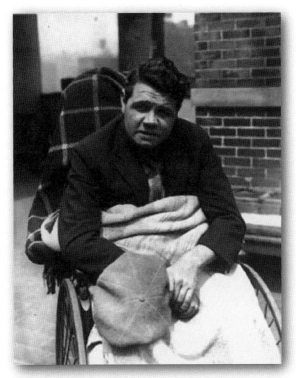

Babe Ruth getting the sunshine atop Saint Vincent's Hospital in New York, May 4, 1925. (©AP Photo)

Back in the day, many hospitals, including my beloved place of residency training, St. Vincent's Hospital in New York City (now demolished to be reborn as high-priced condominiums), had solariums where patients could be exposed to fresh air and sunlight. The healing qualities of sunlight have been known since ancient times.[115] Florence Nightingale, in her book *Notes on Nursing: What It Is, and What It Is Not*, wrote that what patients need most is direct sunlight. "The sun is not only the painter but the sculptor...light has real and tangible effects on the human body."[116] In 1890, Dr. Theobald Palm discovered that sunlight prevented rickets, a bone disease in children. Palm had observed that the disease was virtually absent from children in the Orient but rampant in the cities west and south of England.[117] Early in this century, sunlight, or heliotherapy, was an accepted treatment for tuberculosis, which prompted construction of "heliotherapeutic institutions" in Switzerland where patients were given graduated doses of sun exposure based on the skin's development of erythema (sunburn)—with daily exposure of up to two hours after the skin was tanned.[118]

Vitamin D, "the sunlight vitamin," is produced in your skin after exposure to sunlight, specifically UVB light. Vitamin D produced in the skin or obtained in food or supplements is converted first by the liver to 25 (OH) D; this can be measured in your blood to determine your vitamin D status. The kidneys and many other tissues have vitamin D receptors that will convert 25 (OH) D to a biologically active form.

Because of the association of sun exposure with skin cancer, the use of sunscreens has been widely adapted. The unintended consequence of blocking UVB light is reduced vitamin D production. A sunscreen with an SPF of eight, if applied correctly, will reduce vitamin D production in the skin as much as 95 to 99 percent.[119, 120] Covered in blankets, jacket, and hat, the Babe struck out where his vitamin D level was concerned. He could, however, maintain a healthy vitamin D level by taking a vitamin D supplement or eating sardines, salmon, or other fatty fish that are natural sources of vitamin D. Cod liver oil is a great source but is not particularly easy to take.

Vitamin D status is ascertained by measuring serum 25 (OH) D. A level of less than or equal to 20 ng/ml is considered low by Endocrine Society guidelines and requires treatment. So you think, "I'm a pilot, I'm always outside. How could I be vitamin D deficient?" A recent study of fifty-one internal medicine residents in San Juan, Puerto Rico (a sunny place), found vitamin D deficiency in 43 percent and insufficiency (less than 30 ng/ml) in 45 percent of subjects. The explanation was limited exposure to periods of high sun intensity, limited areas of body exposed, and high BMI.[121] You may spend lots of time outside, but the amount of vitamin D produced in your skin is dependent on how much skin is exposed, whether you use sunscreen, the latitude of your location, the time of day and year, your skin pigmentation, your age, and your BMI.[122] Even in Puerto Rico, it's possible to be vitamin D deficient.

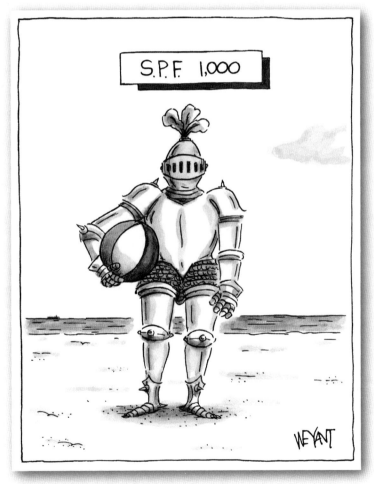

©Christopher Weyant/The New Yorker Collection/The Cartoon Bank.

Although vitamin D is most frequently recommended for bone health—since vitamin D is needed for the absorption of calcium in the gut and for normal skeleton maintenance—this remarkable nutrient is critical for many other body processes. Receptors for vitamin D are present in most tissues, including the brain, breast, and prostate as well as the smooth muscles of blood vessels and macrophages, or the cells involved in arterial plaque production. Vitamin D regulates the expression of about two thousand genes in your cellular DNA by either increasing or decreasing expression of each gene's function. This is probably why low vitamin D levels are associated with increased risks of colon, breast, and prostate cancer as well as cardiovascular disease and autoimmune diseases such as rheumatoid arthritis.[123, 124, 125, 126]

Low vitamin D levels are associated with osteoporosis (low bone calcium), hypertension, metabolic syndrome, atherosclerosis, and elevated serum inflammatory markers. These levels also have direct effects on endothelial cells and the smooth muscle cells of your blood vessels.[127, 128, 129, 130, 131, 132] I have included the following image from a paper by Dr. Paul Norman of the University of Western Australia to drive home this point. Even without understanding every fine point, you can see in this graphic that vitamin D status affects the endothelial cells in arteries, or smooth muscle cells that control vessel function; cardiomyocytes, or the cells of the heart muscle; and various cells that control inflammation. So wouldn't you want to make sure your vitamin D level is optimum?

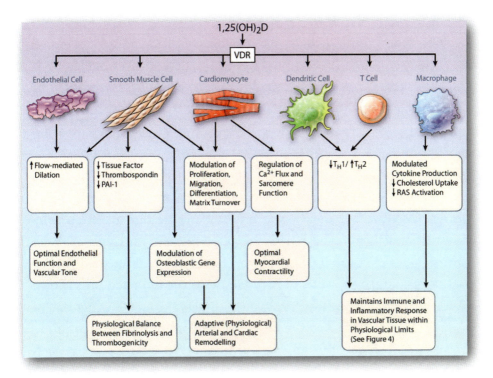

What's optimum? According to the National Institute of Health Office of Dietary Supplements, you are deficient in vitamin D if your serum level is below 30 ng/ml. The Endocrine Society Guidelines define deficiency as less than 20 ng/ml.[133] The Vitamin D Council (www.vitamindcouncil.org), a nonprofit organization that works to educate the public concerning vitamin D, considers levels less than 40 ng/ml deficient and offers the following recommendations regarding 25 (OH) D levels on their website:

- Deficient: 0–40 ng/ml
- Sufficient: 40–80 ng/ml
- High Normal: 80–100 ng/ml
- Undesirable: > 100 ng/ml
- Toxic: > 150 ng/ml

The recommended daily allowance of vitamin D, according to the Food and Nutrition Board of the National Institutes of Health, is 600 IU per day for children and adults up to age seventy, and 800 IU per day for adults over seventy. The Endocrine Society recommends supplement doses for adults of 1,200 to 2,000 IU per day, listing 4,000 IU of vitamin D as the upper tolerable limit for intake. The Vitamin D Council, on the other hand, recommends 5,000 IU per day. The excessive intake of vitamin D in amounts greater than 10,000 IU per day can result in toxicity. Symptoms are nonspecific but are caused by too much calcium in the blood. So many recommendations can be confusing! Have your vitamin D level checked, and discuss with your doctor your supplement needs. Since my profession requires me to work in a room without windows, I routinely take 4,000 IU per day of vitamin D3. Vitamin D works best in combination with magnesium, vitamin K2, zinc, and boron. These nutrients should be readily available in a well-balanced diet or multivitamin supplement.

Sleep Apnea

As you know, the Federal Aviation Administration has mandated that aviation medical examiners screen for obstructive sleep apnea (OSA) as part of the aviation medical exam. OSA is a breathing disorder characterized by episodes of collapse of the upper airway during sleep, resulting in snoring and even complete airway blockage that results in interrupted sleep. People with the condition experience unrestful sleep, awake sleepy, are tired during the daytime, have headaches, and may have difficulty in maintaining attention. If diagnosed, pilots can be medically certified by submitting the required annual status report from their treating physician, along with the results and interpretive report of their most recent sleep study. The FAA's information brochure for pilots states that "people with mild-to-moderate OSA can show performance degradation equivalent to 0.06 to 0.08 percent blood-alcohol levels, which is the measure of legal intoxication in most states." It is not surprising, then, that the FAA would consider this condition a potential safety issue.

The American Academy of Sleep Medicine lists risk factors that should trigger a sleep evaluation: BMI greater than 35, type 2 diabetes, hypertension not responsive to medical treatment, atrial fibrillation, arrhythmias at night, pulmonary hypertension, stroke, congestive heart failure, preoperative evaluation for bariatric surgery, and high-risk driving population (for commercial truck drivers).[134] But OSA is also an independent risk factor for cardiovascular disease. "Apnea" is defined as the cessation of breathing, and if you are not breathing, your blood-oxygen levels drop. You become hypoxic. Intermittent episodes of low blood oxygen and high blood carbon dioxide stimulate factors that contribute to the development sympathetic activation, systemic inflammation, vascular oxidative stress, endothelial dysfunction, increased blood clotting, and metabolic dysregulation that lead to metabolic syndrome.[135, 136, 137, 138, 139, 140]

So, you see, the regulations surrounding sleep apnea are not just oppressive rules from the big government. Sleep apnea has a significant impact on health and should be properly treated. The best way to prevent sleep apnea is to maintain a healthy weight. Avoid nicotine, alcohol, and sleeping medications that will relax the muscles in the back of the throat as these substances can contribute to development of sleep apnea.

CHAPTER 6

Annual Inspection—What Is Your Risk of Heart Disease?

With John Rundback, MD, Director of the Interventional Institute, Holy Name Medical Center

> You don't know what you don't know
> —Old pilot adage

> Never make predictions, especially about the future.
> —Casey Stengel

The goal of most testing is to identify a problem before it occurs so that the appropriate preventive action can be taken. Pilots do a series of checks and tests before flights to identify problems before takeoff, as finding the problem en route is clearly not ideal! The Federal Aviation Regulations mandates an annual aircraft inspection by an FAA-authorized mechanic and additional inspections every hundred hours if the aircraft is used for hire. Systems are checked, oil is changed, and worn components are replaced. The first flight of an airplane just out of annual inspection may uncover problems not identified, or maybe created, during the inspection process. Maybe some of you have had this experience? Most often, these mechanical inspections are done on "asymptomatic" aircraft—that is, performance is great, tires are not worn, and electronics are delivering the goods with no critical potential failure detected.

The problem with medical diagnostic tests is that the accuracy of some tests (the likelihood that an abnormal finding actually means you have a problem) is related to the prevalence of the disease in the sample population. How likely is it to find a mechanical problem in an aircraft with zero hours on the engine and airframe versus the same type of plane with seven thousand hours? Similarly, the likelihood of heart disease in a group of one thousand twenty-year-olds is extremely low. Applying standard testing to this group may result in a number of "false positives"—that is, abnormal results caused not by disease but by other benign conditions that limit the accuracy of the test. If, on the other hand, you test one thousand seventy-year-olds, for whom the likelihood of heart disease is high, a positive result from the same test will carry a much higher likelihood that the result is a *true* positive.

With regard to cardiovascular disease, tests consist of blood analyses and imaging studies. Bear in mind that the results and implications of all these tests are still "up in the air." For example, even though it is well accepted that elevated LDL cholesterol is a risk for subsequent heart attacks and strokes, the guidelines for treatment based upon cholesterol screening changed as recently as 2013. Prior to 2013, doctors would treat patients with an elevated LDL to attempt to reach a target level of less than 100 mg/dl, or less than 70 mg/dl for people at high risk, such as diabetics. However, under the new guidelines of the Blood Cholesterol Expert Panel (previously called the Adult Treatment Panel [ATP] IV), the indications for high- or moderate-intensity statin therapy was changed to identify "patients who would be most likely to benefit" based upon a calculated ten-year risk of cardiovascular events.[141, 142] The reason for this change is that doctors often create guidelines based upon experience rather than on the results of clinical trials; as trial data becomes available, a reanalysis often changes the approach to therapy. For this reason, the new guidelines are less stringent than what existed before, until scientific studies catch up to provide better and proven paradigms for heart disease testing and treatment. Given the issues of testing accuracy and evolving guidelines based on the results of large clinical trials, you may well ask, "Do I need to be tested?" Routine screenings for heart disease are not recommended for people deemed to be at low risk.

ACC/AHA Risk Estimator

The Federal Aviation Administration publishes a Flight Risk Assessment Tool to help identify different levels of flight risk. The tool was developed by reviewing accident data and listing and scoring various crew, operating environment and equipment variables in order to proactively identify potential flight hazards. It is also possible to determine risk for development of heart disease by scoring the parameters that are associated with the development of atherosclerosis. The American Heart Association and the American College of Cardiology have jointly developed a risk calculator that can be accessed online at http://www.cvriskcalculator.com/ or downloaded as an app from iTunes (ASCVD Risk Estimator). The calculator will give you an estimate of your ten-year heart disease risk based on your age, race, gender, total cholesterol, HDL cholesterol, blood pressure, smoking history, and if you are treated for diabetes or high blood pressure. This is a good starting point but does not take into account family history and cannot detect subclinical (not symptomatic) disease.

A risk calculator is a first step in determining if your risk for heart disease is high enough to warrant more expensive and invasive testing. There are several other available risk estimators (some listed below) that you can find online. Emphasis, however, is on the word "estimator." Calculators do not provide clear-cut input as entering waypoints into your GPS would. They take a number of factors and estimate a risk based on population data. General rules do apply, and certain measurable and identifiable health factors can be used to calculate an individual's ten-year risk of cardiovascular events. Everyone's genetic makeup, metabolism, and response to stress is unique, so keep in mind that no mathematical equation regarding health can be 100 percent accurate. For that, we would need to have a Star Trek body scanner!

CARDIOVASCULAR RISK CALCULATORS		
Calculator	Risk Factors Included	Web Site
Framingham Risk Score	Age, sex, total and HDL cholesterol levels, smoking status, systolic blood pressure, and antihypertensive medications.	http://cvdrisk.nhlbi.nih.gov/calculator.asp
SCORE	Age, sex, total-HDL cholesterol ratio, smoking status, and systolic blood pressure	www.heartscore.org/Pages/welcome.aspx
PROCAM*	Age, LDL and HDL cholesterol levels, smoking status, systolic blood pressure, family history, diabetes, and triglyceride levels	http://www.myhealthywaist.org/evaluating-cmr/clinical-tools/index.html
Reynolds Risk Score	Age, HbA1c level†, smoking status, systolic blood pressure, total and HDL cholesterol, hsCRP levels, and parental history of MI at age less than 60 y	www.reynoldsriskscore.org
Pooled Cohort Equation risk calculator	Age, sex, race, total and HDL cholesterol levels, systolic blood pressure, antihypertensive treatment, diabetes and smoking status	www.cardiosource.org/en/Science-And-Quality/Practice-Guidelines-and-Quality-Standards/2013-Prevention-Guideline-Tools.aspx

HbA 1c=hemoglobin A1c; HDL –high density lipoprotein; hcCRP = high-sensitivity C-reactive protein; LDL = low density lipoprotein; MI = myocardial infarction; PROCAM = Prospective Cardiovascular Münster; SCORE = Systemic Coronary Risk Evaluation
*Specific for men; † In women with diabetes

Adapted from "Cardiac Screening with Electrocardiography, Stress Electrocardiography, or Myocardial Perfusion Imaging."[143]

Like all things in flight, the landscape of medical research continues to change. Novel tests are emerging based on genetic analysis of small amounts of blood or cells obtained from swabbing the oral mucosa. In the future, it is indeed conceivable that "tricorders," just like those miraculous scanners in *Star Trek*, will provide an instant and comprehensive evaluation of a person's health and risk of sickness. Technology has already been developed that plugs into an iPhone and periodically or continuously monitors blood sugar in diabetics! However, until these futuristic tools become standardized and mainstream, our assessment of cardiovascular risk—the risk of developing significant heart disease, a stroke, or a heart attack—is based upon a series of somewhat less elegant tests. That being said, let's take a look at what is available now to measure your risk of developing a cardiovascular event:

Physical Examination

Don't forget your regular visits to the doctor. A physical examination allows for the detection of early or new signs of cardiovascular risk. Prior to the actual exam, your doctor will (or should) interview you concerning not only your past medical history and current symptoms (for example, shortness of breath or chest discomfort with exertion, leg pain when walking) but also your family history. Is there heart disease in your immediate family? It's particularly important to know, and to tell your doctor, if someone in your immediate family developed heart disease prior to age fifty. Critical signs of potential problems that can be detected during a physical exam include consistently elevated high blood pressure (also called hypertension), abnormal "whooshing" sounds when listening over the heart or other major arteries (sounds called *bruits*, which indicate a narrowed vessel), an enlarged and pulsatile aorta in the abdomen, or diminished or absent pulses in the arms or feet. With regard to enlargement of the aorta—also called a thoracic (TAA) or abdominal aortic aneurysm

(AAA)—it is important to note that this may also be incidentally discovered during CT scans performed for other reasons!

Hypertension has been labeled the "silent killer"; every ten-point rise in blood pressure is associated with a substantially increased chance of developing a heart attack or stroke. As everyone knows, taking blood pressure involves putting a cuff around the arm, inflating it until it hurts (depending of course upon how sensitive you are), and then slowly deflating it while listening over the artery at the elbow with a stethoscope. Blood pressure is measured as two numbers: the top number, or "systolic" blood pressure, is the pressure level at which the doctor first hears the return of a pulse while deflating the cuff; the lower number, or "diastolic" blood pressure, is when the beating of the artery is no longer heard once the cuff is no longer pressing on the artery. In younger patients, the diastolic blood pressure is a more important measure of heart risk. However, in patients over sixty years old, the systolic number becomes more relevant, as this correlates with the noncompressibility of the arteries. Elevated systolic blood pressure implies that there is generalized atherosclerosis, or "hardening of the arteries," and that the pressure is elevated because the heart is pumping against more resistance.

When measuring blood pressure, two important caveats should be kept in mind. The first is that blood pressure is often higher when a doctor takes it. As I mentioned, this "white coat" hypertension occurs in as many as 20 percent of individuals, and recommendations therefore state that the blood pressure should be measured in both arms after at least a five-minute period of restful sitting. Treatment decisions should be made on the basis of repeated high blood pressure rather than a single measurement. In some cases, it may be necessary to obtain a twenty-four-hour ambulatory blood-pressure measurement. This test, which involves carrying around a small box for twenty-four hours that periodically measures blood pressure during normal activity, is common when evaluating new drugs or devices to treat high blood pressure but is less commonly used in routine practice. The second caveat is that blood pressure may not be the same in both arms; in this case, the pressure in the *higher* arm is more accurate and is the measurement that should be used to determine cardiovascular risk and treatment goals.

Blood Testing
Blood tests that determine the risk of cardiovascular disease, and that potentially change as risks are reduced, are called "biomarkers." The American Heart Association and American College of Cardiology (AHA/ACC) have identified a long list of potential biomarkers, ranging from the common to the obscure. However, some of the more usual and currently available risk-determining blood tests include a measure of the fasting total cholesterol as well as levels of good (HDL) and bad (LDL) cholesterol, hemoglobin A1c, homocysteine and C-reactive protein, and vitamin D.

Cholesterol Screen
As noted earlier, the guidelines for healthy levels of cholesterol have changed over the last few years. Unless you have already been sick or have diabetes, the current recommendations for determining the danger of elevated cholesterol are based upon a ten-year estimated risk of developing coronary artery disease (CAD) exceeding 7.5 percent. Multiple risk calculators are available online. Despite this, the AHA/ACC supports cholesterol treatment for *all* individuals with known CAD regardless of cholesterol levels, patients with an LDL above 190 mg/dl (really high!),

and people with diabetes who are 45 to 75 years old. As for whether elevated cholesterol requires treatment if you don't already have diabetes or CAD, I suggest that unless you are a computer and medical wizard, you should consult with your doctor about your actual risk. A recently validated test called the VAP (Vertical Auto Profile) cholesterol test further measures blood levels of the particle constituents that make up LDL. This test determines the number and size of LDL cholesterol particles and may provide even higher sensitivity for finding the risk of cardiovascular events. It is possible to have a normal LDL-cholesterol level but have a high number of LDL particles. Increased particle number will increase risk of heart disease.

Hemaglobin A1c (HgA1c)
HgA1c level reflects the status of serum blood sugar over the prior three months and is therefore a more reliable measure of potential diabetes than a single fasting blood-sugar test. Normal values are less than 5.7 percent. Values of 5.7 to 6.4 percent indicate "prediabetes," while values of 6.5 percent or greater are consistent with a diagnosis of diabetes. A diagnosis of prediabetes really means that your internal mechanisms for controlling blood glucose are not optimal or are being maxed out by what you eat and by lack of activity; prediabetics are at risk of developing type 2 diabetes and at a higher risk of developing heart disease. For more information regarding prediabetes and diabetes, visit the Joslin Diabetes Center website: www.joslin.org.

> **Type 1 diabetes.** Previously termed juvenile diabetes. Type 1 diabetics need insulin for survival.
> **Type 2 diabetes.** Previously termed adult-onset diabetes. Sugar levels can be controlled with diet or oral medication.

HgA1C is a valuable lab test to help detect the presence of insulin resistance and diabetes, well-established cardiovascular risk factors. There is conflicting data, however, regarding this lab test's accuracy in predicting heart disease risk in people without known diabetes or previously diagnosed heart disease, and a thorough discussion of this would bore you to tears. In summary, a recent collaborative study of almost three hundred thousand participants showed that adding HgA1c to accepted clinical-risk factors yielded very little increase in accuracy in predicting cardiovascular events.[144] Other studies document an 85 percent increased risk of coronary heart disease in men and women with HbA1c levels of 6.0 to 6.5 percent in comparison to individuals with levels of 5 to less than 5 percent.[145] The American College of Cardiology and American Heart Association guidelines do not, at this time, recommend including HbA1c in cardiovascular disease risk assessment. The Canadian Cardiovascular Society, however, does consider elevated HbA1c a risk factor.[146] Transport Canada, the medical certifying agency for Canadian pilots, will request additional testing, including fasting blood glucose, serum lipid profile, and HbA1c, in pilots over age forty with an elevated BMI.

Homocysteine and High-Sensitivity C-Reactive Protein (s-CRP)

These are both "inflammatory markers"—that is, they indicate increased and generalized inflammation in the body. Inflammatory markers are elevated in many diseases, including cardiac disease, infections, and arthritis, and measurements of these markers can be used to determine if any given treatment is effective. In individuals who experience heart disease and stroke, hs-CRP is produced during the process of artery hardening (atherogenesis) and then further aggravates blood-vessel injury and loss of normal function, resulting in blocked arteries.[147]

hs CRP Level	CVD RISK
Less than 1 mg/l	Low
1-3 mg/l	Intermediate
Greater than 3 mg/l	High

A hs-CRP above 3 mg/L is associated with 60 percent excess risk of cardiovascular heart disease compared to risk for levels less than 1 mg/L.[148] Moreover, high hs-CRP individuals with only borderline elevated LDL cholesterol indicate a higher CVD risk than that determined solely on the cholesterol level.[149] Homocysteine is an amino acid (or building block of proteins) that accumulates mostly from eating meat. Elevated homocysteine is often paired with inflammation and is caused by a number of factors, including folate and B-vitamin deficiency, preexisting atherosclerotic disease, and diabetes. Unlike hs-CRP, high homocysteine levels indicate a risk for cardiovascular problems but do not contribute to the process. Vitamin supplementation will lower homocysteine levels, but studies have not demonstrated that this reduces the risk of heart disease.[150, 151] There is, however, evidence that folic acid, vitamins B_6 and B_{12} supplementation do lower homocysteine and the risk of stroke.[152, 153]

Vitamin D

The benefits of a robust serum vitamin D level were discussed in chapter 6. To reiterate, vitamin D is responsible for essential actions not only in the skeletal system but also in just about every organ of our bodies. Vitamin D deficiency is linked to increased risk of cardiovascular disease and high blood pressure (hypertension).[154] The vitamin works directly on the lining of the arteries to stabilize the barrier function of the endothelial cells. (Remember that plaque forms when the endothelium is disrupted.[155]) Direct sunlight, interestingly, has cardiovascular benefits independent of vitamin D, and it is suggested that this may be the result of increased production of nitric oxide, a vasodilator, in the skin triggered by UV-light exposure.[156] I have reprinted here, for your convenience, the vitamin D levels suggested by the Vitamin D Council.

- Deficient: 0–40 ng/ml
- Sufficient: 40–80 ng/ml
- High Normal: 80–100 ng/ml
- Undesirable: > 100 ng/ml
- Toxic: > 150 ng/ml

Imaging

Sophisticated imaging can "look inside" of you and evaluate for signs or conditions that may indicate a higher risk of cardiac events. Radiological tests include computerized axial tomography (CAT or "CT" scans) and ultrasound imaging (sonography). The two principle contemporary CT tests for the heart are coronary calcium scoring, or scanning for calcification on the arteries, and coronary CT angiography, or scanning for blockages in the arteries.

Although not related to cardiovascular risk, CT screening for lung cancers in people with a history of smoking has also been shown to allow the early identification of lung cancer before symptoms develop. This in turn may find cancer while it can still be completely removed and cured by surgery, and large clinical trials have proven that CT screening lowers the risk of lung-cancer death in screened smokers over the age of fifty.

Coronary Calcium Scoring

As you learned in chapter 3, calcium accumulates in arterial plaque. Calcium is easily identified on CT scan, as it appears as dense whiteness on the images. The amount of calcium present in the coronary arteries can be measured by viewing the images of the heart on a CT workstation using a special software program. The resulting sum of the number of sites of coronary artery calcium is the coronary calcium score. A score of 0 means there is no calcified plaque and indicates a very low ten-year risk of coronary heart disease.[157, 158] As the score increases, so does the risk of coronary heart disease. Estimates of risks are shown in the figure below.

SCORE	AMOUNT OF PLAQUE	RISK OF SIGNIFICANT DISEASE
0	NONE	LESS THAN 5%
0-10	MINIMAL	LESS THAT 10%
11-100	MILD	MODERATE
101-400	MODERATE	MODERATE TO HIGH
>400	EXTENSIVE	>90%

This measurement has recently been shown to be one of the strongest predictors of heart-disease risk, and it can increase the accuracy of disease detection in people who, by other risk-scoring methods, were determined to be in low- or intermediate-risk groups.[159, 160] The test is easy, takes only a few minutes to complete, and requires no preparation. Although the test does involve exposure to radiation, current CT scanners administer low doses of radiation. If you have had a CT scan of the neck, chest, or abdomen, ask your doctor if the report documents evidence of arterial calcification. Although there is no specific data to suggest that arterial calcium *outside* the coronary circulation is linked to heart-disease risk, it seems reasonable to assume that if there is calcium in the abdominal arteries, there is likely vascular disease elsewhere.

Coronary CT Angiography (CCTA)

In the past, the most direct way of imaging coronary arteries was with cardiac catheterization, an invasive procedure that involves placing a catheter in an artery in the groin or wrist and advancing the catheter into the heart and coronary arteries. Dye is then injected directly into the arteries, and pictures are recorded. Although considered a routine procedure with low risk, this is an invasive test that is reserved for patients at high risk for coronary artery disease.

There is, however, a noninvasive method to image the coronary arteries with CT scan. This technique has been used for the last ten years, and with improvements in CT technology, radiation dose has decreased and image quality has markedly improved. A radiology dye is injected into an arm vein, and images of the heart are obtained in synchronization with the heartbeat. Depending on the CT scanner being used, you may be given medication to lower your heart rate to a range that will optimize imaging and reduce artifacts that are created by motion. The benefit of this technique over the more invasive cardiac catheterization is that the whole vessel wall, not just the lumen, can be evaluated. This means that both calcified and noncalcified plaques as well as the degree of narrowing can be assessed. The limitation, even with most advanced CT scanners, is that small vessels are not seen as adequately as with direct cardiac catheterization. CCTA is used as a problem solver in patients with intermediate risk of heart disease who have yielded equivocal results in routine exercise stress tests. It is also used in emergency departments to evaluate patients with atypical chest pain, to evaluate the patency of coronary artery bypass grafts, to investigate increasing symptoms in patients with otherwise normal test results, and to evaluate patients with possible congenital coronary artery anomalies. For the pilots who do have a myocardial infarction, stent placement, or bypass surgery, the FAA will not yet accept this test in lieu of a cardiac catheterization in the initial post event submission for medical certification.

Carotid Ultrasound

The intima and media are the inner and middle (muscular) linings of the arteries, and the thickness of these layers can be easily measured using ultrasound imaging of the carotid arteries that are superficially located in the neck. The rationale for this test is that the increased thickness of the layers beneath the lining of the carotid artery is a measure of developing plaque and therefore might be a method to detect subclinical (i.e., not symptomatic) vascular disease.[161] Carotid intimal media thickness (CIMT) varies with age, and the upper-limit normal CIMT is 1.5 mm. Because this is an easy test to perform and because the ultrasound scanners used to perform the test are relatively low cost, this procedure is becoming widely available. The CIMT is best utilized in evaluating patients who are considered at intermediate risk by normal and more traditional algorithms, namely, the Framingham Risk Score. This score looks at age, diabetic status, total and HDL cholesterol, smoking, systolic blood pressure, and gender to calculate the risk of heart attack over the next ten years. In patients with an intermediate risk (10–20 percent ten-year risk of heart attack), an elevated CIMT is useful to guide your physician to do other more detailed tests, such as coronary stress testing or echocardiography.

Vascular Endothelial Dysfunction

The endothelium is a single cell layer lining the inside of blood vessels that is biologically very active, secreting multiple hormones to control blood flow, or "tone," under different environmental circumstances. Endothelial function testing is performed by performing ultrasound over the artery at the elbow; it looks for relaxation of the artery after overinflation and the release of a blood-pressure cuff. Under normal circumstances, the artery should relax, or dilate fully, to maximize blood flow back to the hand that has been deprived of flow for several minutes. This ability for the vessel dilate is controlled by the release of the local hormone (also called a cytokine) named nitrous oxide from the endothelium. Endothelial function testing showing a reduced relaxation of the vessel implies dysfunction.[162, 163] Interestingly, although this is measured in the arm, impaired endothelial function is often systemic (i.e., affecting all arteries in the body) and includes the coronary arteries. Therefore, it makes sense that an abnormal endothelial function test has been repeatedly shown to be associated with a higher cardiovascular risk. Unfortunately, the test readings can be influenced by many factors, including stress, medications, recent meals, room temperature, and viral illness. For this reason, there are ongoing efforts to standardize the test so that it can be reliably used in clinical practice.

Ankle-Brachial Index

There are many other tests in practice and development that are designed to accurately determine someone's risk of a heart attack or stroke so that appropriate treatment can be started early. One of the least frequently utilized, and yet easiest to perform and highly predictive, is a measurement of ankle-brachial index, or ABI. In normal adults, since the arteries are a closed system, the pressure in an artery at any location in the body should be roughly the same. However, for individuals who have peripheral artery disease (PAD), hardening of the arteries causes narrowing of the blood flow to one or both legs. As a result, a measurement of the blood pressure in the ankle *beyond* the point of this narrowing will be lower than blood pressure measured in the arm—similar to a kink in a fuel line! This ratio—the ankle blood pressure compared to the arm blood pressure—is the ABI. Measuring the ABI is a simple, painless, and highly reliable measure of premature heart attack, stroke, and early mortality.[164] ABI testing is recommended by the AHA/ACC for any patient who has absent pulses in the feet or symptoms compatible with PAD (for instance, pain when walking that is relieved by standing rest), patients over the age of fifty who smoke or have diabetes, or patients over the age of seventy regardless of risk factors. Up to 40 percent of patients with PAD die from cardiac events within five years of diagnosis, and there is a linear correlation between the severity of PAD (how low the ABI is) and this five-year risk.

Genetic Testing

Clearly there is a familial, hereditary risk of heart disease; this is common knowledge. For more than a decade, genetic testing has measured multiple genes and the proteins they produce to estimate a person's susceptibility to cardiac events. There are hundreds if not thousands of "candidate" genes that can be measured.[165] However, there is much controversy about the value of genetic testing, mostly for two reasons: First of all, the actual risk of a heart attack is determined not only by a person's genetic code but also by their environmental exposure, habits (smoking in particular), exercise level, and diet. Second, since gene testing therefore does not necessarily predict an unavoidable future heart attack or stroke, there is tremendous ethical concern about how someone might react to knowing his or her potential genetic risk.[166] Despite this, since the human genome is now fully mapped, it is only a matter of time until near-noninvasive tests (maybe even a swab of oral mucosa) will be used to perform reliable gene and protein testing not only to determine risk but also to identify the best ways to avoid it. Advances of this nature are almost inevitable and may even occur in time to help the next generation!

Two well-studied genetically linked conditions that result in a significant increased risk for premature cardiovascular disease and stroke are familial hypercholesterolemia (very high cholesterol and LDL-C) and familial hypertriglyceridemia (very high triglycerides). Individuals with familial hypercholesterolemia may have abnormally deposited cholesterol around the joints (xanthomas) or in the eyes. About one in two hundred people have this disorder, and many go undiagnosed. This is a treatable disease that can be detected by simple cholesterol screening and evaluation of family history. For more information visit the FH Foundation website at http//: www.thefhfoundation.org.

Exercise Stress Testing and Myocardial Perfusion Imaging

An exercise stress test, termed by the FAA as graded exercise stress test (GXT), is a method to determine your heart's performance during increasing levels of physical activity; you walk on a treadmill while an electrocardiogram (ECG) monitors changes in your heart as the treadmill increases in speed and incline. An ECG is a graphic depiction of the electrical impulses that are produced in the heart with each heartbeat. Each heartbeat is initiated by an electrical system embedded in the heart muscle. The picture below illustrates these pathways, which originate in the sinoatrial node and then travel to the rest of the heart, and an example of the ECG that is produced. When these signals are disrupted, arrhythmias, such as atrial fibrillation, will occur. A resting ECG, required once a year for airline and commercial pilots, will detect disruptions in the electrical pathways and reveal abnormal heart rhythm or evidence of prior heart attck.

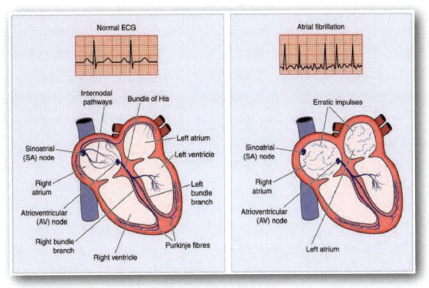

©Blamb/Shutterstock.com

Under conditions of exercise and increasing heart rate, coronary blood flow increases to meet the heart muscle's demand for more oxygen. If there is inadequate flow to a region of the muscles, this is reflected in changes in the ECG tracing. Accuracy of this test depends on several factors, including the level of exercise achieved.

To improve accuracy in detection of coronary artery stenosis, the GXT is combined with heart imaging and myocardial perfusion imaging (MPI). For this test, a small amount of a radioactive chemical (radiopharmaceutical) that deposits in the heart muscle is administered intravenously prior to exercising, and images of the heart are acquired. A second injection of the same agent is administered while the patient is on the treadmill at the time of peak exercise, and a second set of images is obtained. In a normal exam of a healthy person, the myocardial distribution of radiopharmaceutical appears the same at rest as during stress. If there is coronary artery narrowing, the stress images will show a defect in the heart muscle that is not apparent on the rest images. This is because a healthy, unaffected heart will, during exercise and related increased coronary blood flow, experience increased myocardial uptake—displayed clearly by increased delivery of the radiopharmaceutical. A diseased coronary cannot increase blood flow, and consequently, the amount of radiopharmaceutical delivered to the heart muscle will be less. The combination of normal rest images and abnormal stress images indicates the presence of a significantly narrowed coronary artery and myocardial ischemia.

If you have had a heart attack, the region of damage will be abnormal on both the rest and stress images. In this case, ischemia, if present, may occur at the margins of the infarct and will be seen as areas of decreased uptake on stress images compared to the rest images. The FAA requires MPI stress testing on alternate years for pilots requesting First and Second Class Medical Special Issuance.

CHAPTER 7

Conclusion

> When you are young and healthy, it never
> occurs to you that in a single second
> your whole life could change.
> —Annette Funicello

> Be careful about reading health books.
> You may die of a misprint.
> —Mark Twain

Heart disease is not the result of any one particular food, activity, or inherited predisposition. I trust that by reading this book and understanding the complex mechanisms involved in the development of atherosclerosis—and, ultimately, heart disease—you will be motivated to adopt positive lifestyle changes, including improving diet and avoiding inactivity; by recognizing sources of chronic stress, you can adopt stress-reduction techniques. Health-promoting choices, along with accurate screening for heart disease, will help keep you in the left seat for life. But all this requires commitment and self-control.

My first eight years of schooling were spent in Visitation Academy of the Sacred Heart in Bay Ridge, Brooklyn, an all-girls private grammar school run by the Sisters of the Visitation, a semicloistered religious order. "Semicloistered" meant that our parents could communicate with the sisters only though a wooden lattice darkened by a translucent black cloth. Sounds medieval, doesn't it? We were taught obedience and self-control from an early age with the threat of being given a *demerit*, which was an orange card with "DEMERIT" written on it in perfect script. The student was to take this dreaded card home and have their parent sign it. Perhaps this approach is a far cry from Dr. Benjamin Spock's child-rearing principles, but the ability to control impulses is not a bad thing, and in fact, it might give you the few seconds necessary to reconsider whether you really need that last slice of pepperoni pizza, not to mention other more damaging choices.

We are faced with choices every day. Sometimes a decision, like choosing a direction in a forked road, will place you on a path that may make it almost impossible to return to what would have been a better place. Taking the time to learn about how your body systems work and what is required for optimum functioning will have far-reaching effects.

The price of health care in the United States, both for the government and the consumer, continues to increase. My observation, as a hospital-based radiologist, is that many people simply lack the basic knowledge needed to take care of themselves. There is a vast difference between a true medical emergency and an upset stomach from constipation. I often think we should staff the emergency departments with wise grandmothers. Not every ill requires a pill. Many "illnesses" can be prevented or improved with the right food choices and adequate activity.

To take this a step further, I think that if we considered investing in our health as in IRA or pension plans, many of us might have a very different approach to health. Think about the downstream financial benefits of maintaining a healthy lifestyle. What will it cost you in the future to deal with the expense of type 2 diabetes or coronary heart disease? What does it cost you now to turn around poor eating habits, reduce time sitting, and learn to manage stress?

There are thousands of books, websites, and videos that purport to offer the best exercise or diet or health program, but the best advice I think I was ever given was from my grandmother, Ann, who was still wearing designer high heels well into her eighties. She said, "You have to force yourself!"

Checklist

1. Limit the amount of sitting, or break up periods of sitting. Invest in a step monitor.
2. Eat a Mediterranean-style diet. Limit or eliminate intake of sugar. Read labels.
3. Identify stressors in your life, and incorporate mechanisms to break them.
4. Understand your family-health history. You may have inherited a predisposition for certain diseases, which could require additional preventive measures.
5. Find a doctor you trust, who listens to you.
6. Have your vitamin D level checked.
7. Discuss with your doctor the benefits of testing based on your specific risk factors. Tests could include routine evaluations of fasting blood glucose, cholesterol screenings with VAP, and tests for inflammatory markers.
8. Knowledge is power. Be an informed consumer of the medical industry.

Recommendations

Devices

1. **Fitbit.** https://www.fitbit.com. The step tracker that I use. I have also invested in the Fitbit scale, which tracks weight and body fat.
2. **Xiser.** https://xiser.com. Portable stepper for high-intensity training. I have one at home and one at work. It's a little pricey but extremely well made.
3. **RESPeRATE.** www.resperate.com. An affordable device that is FDA approved to reduce blood pressure by controlling breathing.

Websites and Apps

1. **https://www.myfitnesspal.com.** Excellent app and website to track food intake and exercise. It includes exercise suggestions as well as great recipes.
2. **ASCVD Risk Estimator, iPhone and Android app.** American College of Cardiology/American Heart Association tool to

help estimate ten-year risk of cardiovascular disease. I suggest that you use this with your doctor's input.

3. **https://www.consumerlab.com.** This is not a free website. For a membership fee of thirty-nine dollars for one year, you have access to nutritional-supplement reviews, quality ratings, and brand comparisons. Membership also includes an e-newsletter as well as alerts and warnings concerning products tested.
4. **www.vitamindcouncil.org.** The Vitamin D Council provides information about vitamin D and publishes news regarding related research.
5. **www.mayoclinic.org.** Excellent website for information about health issues as well as drugs and supplements.
6. **www.webmed.com.** Another easy-to-navigate website for research on specific health concerns, recommendations for healthy lifestyles, and information about drugs and supplements.
7. **www.drweil.com.** My mentor, Dr. Andrew Weil, offers a library of health information on this website. Included on this site is a "vitamin advisor," which will give you recommendations for specific supplements based on your answers to questions regarding your current health status.
8. **http://lpi.oregonstate.edu/.** The Linus Pauling Institute website provides research-backed information regarding vitamins and supplements. Some of the information presented is not for the academically faint of heart.
9. **www.vitalchoice.com.** A source for ordering high-quality organic foods. Carries sustainable wild-caught salmon as well as other fish products.

Books

1. Daniel, Kaayla T. *The Whole Soy Story*. Washington, DC: New Trends Publishing, 2005. My opinion: too much processed soy just isn't good. This book will tell you why.
2. Gaynor, Mitchell L. *The Gene Therapy Plan*. New York: Viking Penguin, 2015. This book explains ways to change expression of your genes with diet and lifestyle to promote health and prevent disease.
3. Kellman, Raphael. *The Microbiome Diet*. Boston: Da Capo Press, 2014. More information about how to feed your gut bacteria.
4. Low Dog, Tieraona. *Healthy at Home*. Washington, DC: National Geographic, 2014. You don't need medicine for every ailment. This is a wonderful source of home remedies for minor illnesses.
5. Mercola, Joseph. *Sweet Deception*. Tennessee: Nelson Books, 2006. Read this, and you might avoid that next diet soda.
6. Oz, Michael. *You, The Owner's Manual*. New York: Harper Collins, 2005. The best source for learning about how your body works. Any book by Dr. Oz is well worth the read.
7. Perlmutter, David. *Grain Brain*. New York: Little, Brown and Company, 2013. A comprehensive explanation about inflammation and degenerative disease, specifically the effects of inflammation on the brain.
8. Schwartz, Erika. *Don't Let Your Doctor Kill You*. New York: Post Hill Press, 2015. Erika and I were classmates in medical school and have identical attitudes regarding the practice of medicine. With examples of both the best and the worst medicine, Erika provides a roadmap for patients and physicians alike to

work together to provide safer, compassionate, and careful health care. A must-read for everyone.
9. Sonnenburg, Justin, and Erica Sonnenburg. *The Good Gut.* New York: Penguin Random House, 2015. If you want to learn more about your microbiome, this is the book.
10. Vernikos, Joan. *Sitting Kills.* Fresno: Quill Driver Books, 2011. An easy, entertaining read by a former NASA scientist that will definitely keep you off the couch.
11. Weil, Andrew. *Spontaneous Happiness.* New York: Little, Brown and Company, 2013. I can recommend any and all of Dr. Weil's books. This one details his personal approach to balancing emotional life.

About The Author

Jacqueline Brunetti, MD, is the Director of Radiology at Holy Name Medical Center in Teaneck, New Jersey; an Associate Professor of Clinical Radiology, part-time, at New York—Presbyterian Medical Center, Columbia University College of Physicians and Surgeons; and a Senior FAA Aviation Medical Examiner.

She is board certified in radiology, nuclear medicine, nuclear radiology, and integrative medicine; maintains membership in numerous professional organizations; and serves as a consultant to the Medical Devices Advisory Committee of the FDA.

Dr. Brunetti holds a private pilot's license with logged flight hours in both single-engine and turboprop airplanes. An FAA-designated aviation medical examiner for more than twenty years, she has been a senior medical examiner for fifteen years. She is also a certified human intervention medical sponsor, trained to help evaluate pilots with substance abuse, depression, and other psychiatric issues.

Dr. Brunetti has appeared on radio and television broadcasts including CNN, NJ Channel 12, WABC, and WOR.

NOTES

1. C. K. Meador, "The Last Well Person," *New England Journal of Medicine (NEJM)* 330, no. 6 (1994): 440–41.
2. S. Evans and S. A. Radcliffe, "The Annual Incapacitation Rate of Commercial Pilots," *Aviation, Space, and Environmental Medicine* 83, no. 1 (2012): 42–49.
3. S. R. Mohler and C. F. Booze, "US Fatal General Aviation Accidents Due to Cardiovascular Incapacitation: 1974–75," *Aviation, Space and Environmental Medicine* 49, no. 10 (1978): 1225–28.
4. S. Di Francescomarino, A. Sciartelli, V. Di Valerio et al., "The Effect of Physical Exercise on Endothelial Function," *Sports Medicine* 39, no. 10 (2009): 797–812.
5. M. Ross and W. Pawlina, *Histology: A Text and Atlas* (Philadelphia: Wolters Kluwer LWW, 2011), 409–30.
6. B. M. Scirica and C. P. Cannon, "Treatment of Elevated Cholesterol," *Circulation* 111, no. 21 (2005): e360–63.
7. D. Lu and G. S. Kassab, "Role of Shear Stress and Stretch in Vascular Mechanobiology," *Journal of the Royal Society Interface* 8, no. 63 (2011): 1379–85.
8. C. Zaragoza, S. Marquez et al., "Endothelial Mechanosensors of Shear Stress as Regulators of Atherogenesis," *Current Opinion in Lipidology* 23, no. 5 (2012): 446–52.
9. I. Tabas, K. J. Williams et al., "Subendothelial Lipoprotein Retention as the Initiating Process in Atherosclerosis: Update and Therapeutic Implications," *Circulation* 116, no. 16 (2007): 1832–44.
10. F. R. Maxfield and I. Tabas, "Role of Cholesterol and Lipid Organization in Disease," *Nature* 438, no. 7068 (2005): 36–45.

11. J. Kaur, "A Comprehensive Review on Metabolic Syndrome," *Cardiovascular Research and Practice* 2014, Article ID 943162, (2014): 21 pages.
12. Ibid.
13. J. A. Kim, M. Montagnani, K. K. Koh et al., "Reciprocal Relationships between Insulin Resistance and Endothelial Dysfunction," *Circulation* 113, no. 15 (2006): 1888–1904.
14. V. T. Samuel and G. I. Shulman, "Integrating Mechanisms for Insulin Resistance: Common Threads and Missing Links," *Cell* 148, no. 5 (2012): 852–71.
15. K. G. Alberti, P. Zimmet, and J. Shaw, "Metabolic Syndrome—A New Worldwide Definition. A Consensus Statement from the International Diabetes Federation," *Diabetic Medicine* 23, no. 5 (2006): 469–80.
16. D. E. Laaksonen, H. M. Lakka, L. K. Niskanen et al., "Metabolic Syndrome and the Development of Diabetes Mellitus: Application and Validation of Recently Suggested Definitions of the Metabolic Syndrome in a Prospective Cohort Study," *American Journal of Epidemiology* 156, no. 11 (2002): 1070–77.
17. C. Lorenzo, M. Okoloise, K. Williams et al., "The Metabolic Syndrome as Predictor of Type 2 Diabetes," *Diabetes Care* 26, no. 11 (2003): 3153–59.
18. P. W. F. Wilson, R. B. D'Agostino, H. Parise et al., "Metabolic Syndrome as Precursor of Cardiovascular Disease and Type 2 Diabetes Mellitus," *Circulation* 112, no. 20 (2005): 3066–72.
19. J. A. Shin, J. H. Lee, S. Y. Lim et al., "Metabolic Syndrome as the Predictor of Type 2 Diabetes, and Its Clinical Interpretations and Usefulness," *Journal of Diabetes Investigation* 4, no. 4 (2013): 334–43.

20. H. Sabour, A. N. Javidan, N. Ranjbarnovin et al., "Cardiometabolic Risk Factors in Iranians with Spinal Cord Injury: Analysis by Injury-Related Variables," *Journal of Rehabilitation Research and Development* 50, no. 5 (2013): 635–42.
21. A. Libin, E. A. Tinsley, M. S. Nash et al., "Cardiometabolic Risk Clustering in Spinal Cord Injury: Results of Exploratory Factor Analysis," *Topics in Spinal Cord Injury Rehabilitation* 19, no. 3 (2013): 183–94.
22. P. Flank, K. Wahman, R. Levi et al., "Prevalence of Risk Factors for Cardiovascular Disease Stratified by Body Mass Index Categories in Patients with Wheelchair-Dependent Paraplegia after Spinal Cord Injury," *Journal of Rehabilitation Medicine* 44, no. 5 (2012): 440–43.
23. K. Wahman, M. S. Nash, J. E. Lewis et al., "Cardiovascular Disease Risk and the Need for Prevention after Paraplegia Determined by Conventional Multifactorial Risk Models: The Stockholm Spinal Cord Injury Study," *Journal of Rehabilitation Medicine* 43, no. 3 (2011): 237–42.
24. M. D. Nelson, L. M. Widman, and C. M. McDonald, "Metabolic Syndrome in Adolescents with Spinal Cord Injury," *Journal of Spinal Cord Medicine* 30, Suppl 1 (2007): S127–S139.
25. J. J. Cragg, V. K. Noonan, A. Krassioukov et al., "Cardiovascular Disease in Spinal Cord Injury," *Neurology* 81, no. 8 (2013): 723–28.
26. H. Sandler and J. Vernikos, *Inactivity: Physiological Effects* (Orlando: Academic Press, Inc., 1986): 11–95.
27. G. Clement and A. Bukley, *Artificial Gravity* (Hawthorne: Microcosm Press; New York: Springer, 2007): 137–159.
28. J. Vernikos, *Sitting Kills, Moving Heals* (Fresno: Quill Driver Books, 2011).

29. J. R. Zierath and J. A. Hawley, "Skeletal Muscle Fiber Type: Influence on Contractile and Metabolic Properties," *PLOS Biology* 2, no. 10 (2004): 1523–27.
30. H. O. Tikkanen, E. Hamalainen, and M. Harkonen, "Significance of Skeletal Muscle Properties on Fitness, Long-Term Physical Training, and Serum Lipids," *Atherosclerosis* 142, no. 2 (1999): 367–78.
31. R. H. Fitts, D. R. Riley, and J. J. Widrick, "Functional and Structural Adaptations of Skeletal Muscle to Microgravity," *Journal of Experimental Biology* 2014 (2001): 3201–08.
32. D. Hart, "Is Adipocyte Differentiation the Default Lineage for Mesenchymal Stem/Progenitor Cells after Loss of Mechanical Loading? A Perspective from Space Flight and Model Systems," *Journal of Biomedical Science and Engineering* 7, no. 10 (2014): 799–808.
33. O. Hamdy, S. Porramatikul, and E. Al-Ozari, "Metabolic Obesity: The Paradox between Visceral and Subcutaneous Fat," *Current Diabetes Reviews* 2, no. 4 (2006): 367–73.
34. H. Kwon and J. E. Pessin, "Adipokines Mediate Inflammation and Insulin Resistance," *Frontiers in Endocrinology* 4, Article 71 (2013): 1–13.
35. T. Romacho, M. Elsen, D. Rohrborn et al., "Adipose Tissue and Its Role in Organ Crosstalk," *Acta Physiologica* 210, no. 4 (2014): 733–53.
36. A. R. G. Proenca, R. A. L. Sertie, A. C. Oliveira et al., "New Concepts in White Adipose Tissue Physiology," *Brazilian Journal of Medical and Biological Research* 47, no. 3 (2014): 192–205.
37. A. Shezad, W. Iqbal, O. Shehzad et al., "Adiponectin: Regulation of Its Production and Its Role in Human Diseases," *Hormones* 11, no. 1 (2012): 8–20.

38. A. D. Kriketos, S. K. Gan, A. M. Poynten et al., "Exercise Increases Adiponectin Levels and Insulin Sensitivity in Humans," *Diabetes Care* 27, no. 2 (2004): 629–30.
39. K. A. Simpson and M. A. Singh, "Effects of Exercise on Adiponectin: A Systematic Review," *Obesity* 16, no. 2 (2008): 241–56.
40. M. C. Passos and M. C. Goncalves, "Regulation of Insulin Sensitivity by Adiponectin and Its Receptors in Response to Exercise," *Hormone and Metabolic Research* 46, no. 9 (2014): 603–08.
41. D. Y. Kim, B. D. Seo, and D. J. Kim, "Effect of Walking Exercise on Changes in Cardiorespiratory Fitness, Metabolic Syndrome Markers, and High-Molecular-Weight Adiponectin in Obese Middle-Aged Women," *Journal of Physical Therapy Science* 26, no. 11 (2014): 1723–27.
42. C. J. Huang, C. F. Kwok, C. H. Chou et al., "The Effect of Exercise on Lipid Profiles and Inflammatory Markers in Lean Male Adolescents: A Prospective Interventional Study," *Journal of Investigative Medicine* 63, no. 1 (2015): 29–34.
43. C. Brandt and B. Pedersen, "The Role of Exercise-Induced Myokines in Muscle Homeostasis and the Defense against Chronic Diseases," *Journal of Biomedicine and Biotechnology* 2010 (2010): 520258.
44. B. Strasser and D. Pesta, "Resistance Training for Diabetes Prevention and Therapy: Experimental Findings and Molecular Mechanisms," *BioMed Research International* 2013 (2013): 805217.
45. J. Myers, "Exercise and Cardiovascular Health," *Circulation* 107 (2003): e2–e5.
46. B. R. Stephens, K. Granados, T. W. Zderic et al., "Effects of 1 day of Inactivity on Insulin Action in Healthy Men and Women: Interaction with Energy Intake," *Metabolism* 60, no. 7 (2011): 941–49.

47. B. M. F. M. Duvivier, N. C. Schaper, M. A. Bremers et al., "Minimal Intensity Physical Activity (Standing and Walking) of Longer Duration Improves Insulin Action and Plasma Lipids More than Shorter Periods of Moderate to Vigorous Exercise (Cycling) in Sedentary Subjects When Energy Expenditure is Comparable," *PLOS ONE* 8 (2013): e55542.
48. D. W. Dunstan, B. A. Kingwell, R. Larsen et al., "Breaking Up Prolonged Sitting Reduces Postprandial Glucose and Insulin Responses," *Diabetes Care* 35, no. 5 (2012): 976–83.
49. C. Tudor-Locke, C. L. Craig, J. P. Thyfault et al., "A Step-Defined Lifestyle Index: < 5,000 steps/day," *Applied Physiology, Nutrition, and Metabolism* 38, no. 2 (2013): 100–14.
50. C. Tudor-Locke, C. L. Craig, Y. Aoyagi et al., "How Many Steps/Day Are Enough? For Adults," *International Journal of Behavioral Nutrition and Physical Activity* 28 (2011): 79.
51. P. Jennersjo, J. Ludvigsson, T. Lanne et al., "Pedometer-Determined Physical Activity is Linked to Low Systemic Inflammation and Low Arterial Stiffness in Type 2 Diabetes," *Diabetic Medicine* 29, no. 9 (2012): 1119–25.
52. W. L. Haskell, I. M. Lee, R. R. Pate et al., "Physical Activity and Public Health: Updated Recommendation for Adults for the American College of Sports Medicine and the American Heart Association," *Medicine and Science in Sports and Exercise* 39, no. 8 (2007): 1423–34.
53. W. L. Westcott, "Resistance Training Is Medicine: Effects of Strength Training on Health," *Current Sports Medicine Reports* 11, no. 4 (2012): 209–16.
54. N. K. LeBrasseur, K. Walsh, and Z. Arany, "Metabolic Benefits of Resistance Training and Fast Glycoluting Skeletal Muscle,"

American Journal of Physiology—Endocrinology and Metabolism 300, no. 1 (2011): E3–E10.

55. R. Norris, D. Carroll, and R. Cochrane, "The Effects of Aerobic and Anaerobic Training on Fitness, Blood Pressure and Psychological Stress and Well-being," *Journal of Psychosomatic Research* 34, no. 4 (1990): 367–75.

56. N. Norvell and D. Belles, "Psychological and Physical Benefits of Circuit Weight Training in Law Enforcement Personnel," *Journal of Consulting and Clinical Psychology* 61, no. 3 (1993): 520–27.

57. J. C. Strickland and M. A. Smith, "The Anxiolytic Effects of Resistance Exercise," *Frontiers in Psychology* 5 (2014): 753.

58. C. A. Slentz, L. A. Bateman, L. H. Willis et al., "Effects of Aerobic vs. Resistance Training on Visceral and Liver Fat Stores, Liver Enzymes, and Insulin Resistance by HOMA in Overweight Adults from STRRIDE AT/RT," *American Journal of Physiology-Endocrinology and Metabolism* 301, no. 5 (2011): E1033–E1039.

59. A. McCann, *Starving America* (New York: George H. Doran Company, 1912).

60. A. M. Mayer, "Historical Changes in the Mineral Content of Fruits and Vegetables," *British Food Journal* 99, no. 6 (1997): 207–11.

61. D. R. Davis, M. D. Epp, and H. D. Riordan, "Changes in USDA Food Composition Data for 43 Garden Crops, 1950 to 1999," *Journal of the American College of Nutrition* 23, no. 6 (2004): 669–82.

62. S. M. Wunderlich, C. Feldman, S. Kane et al., "Nutritional Quality of Organic, Conventional, and Seasonally Grown Broccoli Using Vitamin C as a Marker," *International Journal of Food Sciences and Nutrition* 59, no. 1 (2008): 43–5.

63. D. R. Davis, "Declining Fruit and Vegetable Nutrient Composition: What is the Evidence?" *HortScience* 44, no. 1 (2009): 15–19.

64. J. Reeves, "The Rise and Fall of Food Minerals," *Nutrition and Health* 20, no. 3–4 (2011): 209–29.
65. A. Keys, "Coronary Heart Disease in Seven Countries". *Circulation* 41, no. 1 (1970): 186–95.
66. A. Keys, C. Aravanis, H. Blackburn et al., *Seven Countries: A Multivariate Analysis of Death and Coronary Artery Disease* (Cambridge: Harvard University Press, 1980).
67. A. Bach-Faig, E. M. Berry, D. Lairon et al., "Mediterranean Diet Pyramid Today. Science and Cultural Updates," *Public Health Nutrition* 14, Special Issue 12A (2011): 2274–84.
68. R. Estruch, E. Ros, J. Salas-Salvado et al., "Primary Prevention of Cardiovascular Disease with a Mediterranean Diet," *New England Journal of Medicine* 368, no. 14 (2013): 1279–90.
69. A. C. Grandjean and N. R. Grandjean, "Dehydration and Cognitive Performance," *Journal of the American College of Nutrition* 26, Suppl 5 (2007): 549S–554S.
70. D. Benton, "Dehydration Influences Mood and Cognition: A Plausible Hypothesis?" *Nutrients* 3, no. 5 (2011): 555–73.
71. S. K. Riebl and B. M. Davy, "The Hydration Equation: Update on Water Balance and Cognitive Performance," *American College of Sports Medicine's Health and Fitness Journal* 17, no. 6 (2013): 21–28.
72. N. A. Masento, M. Golightly, D. T. Field et al., "Effects of Hydration on Cognitive Performance and Mood," *British Journal of Nutrition* 111, no. 10 (2014): 1841–52.
73. I. Salim, J. Al Suwadi, W. Ghadban et al., "Impact of Religious Ramadan Fasting on Cardiovascular Disease: Systematic Review of the Literature," *Current Medical Research and Opinion* 29, no. 4 (2013): 343–54.

74. M. Nematy, M. Alinezhad-Namaght, M. M. Rashed et al., "Effects of Ramadan Fasting on Cardiovascular Factors: A Prospective Observational Study," *Nutrition Journal* 11, no. 1 (2012): 69.
75. B. Yousefi, Z. Faghfoori, N. Samadi et al., "The Effects of Ramadan Fasting on Endothelial Function in Patients with Cardiovascular Disease," *European Journal of Clinical Nutrition* 68, no. 7 (2014): 835–39.
76. S. Brandhorst, I. Y. Choi, C. W. Cheng et al., "A Periodic Diet that Mimics Fasting Promotes Multi-System Regeneration, Enhanced Cognitive Performance, and Healthspan," *Cell Metabolism* 22, no. 1 (July 7, 2015): 86–99.
77. J. E. Brown, M. Mosley, and S. Aldred, "Intermittent Fasting: A Dietary Intervention for Prevention of Diabetes and Cardiovascular Disease?" *British Journal of Diabetes and Vascular Disease* 13, no. 2 (2013): 68–72.
78. A. Cherkas and S. Golota, "An Intermittent Exhaustion of the Pool of Glycogen in Human Organism as a Simple Universal Health Promoting Mechanism," *Medical Hypotheses* 82, no. 3 (March 2014): 387–89.
79. D. Ornish, L. W. Scherwitz, R. S. Doody et al., "Effects of Stress Management Training and Dietary Changes in Treating Ischemic Heart Disease," *Journal of the American Medical Association* 249, no. 1 (1983): 54–59.
80. K. L. Gould, D. Ornish, L. Scherwitz et al., "Changes in Myocardial Perfusion Abnormalities by Positron Emission Tomography after Long-Term Intense Risk Factor Modification," *Journal of the American Medical Association* 274, no. 11 (1995): 894–901.

81. D. Ornish, L. W. Scherwitz, J. H. Billings et al., "Intensive Lifestyle Changes for Reversal of Coronary Heart Disease," *Journal of the American Medical Association* 280, no. 23 (1998): 2001–07.
82. J. J. Daubenmier, G. Weidner, M. D. Sumner et al., "The Contribution of Changes in Diet and Exercise, and Stress Management to Changes in Coronary Risk in Women and Men in the Multisite Cardiac Lifestyle Intervention Program," *Annals of Behavioral Medicine* 33, no. 1 (2007): 57–68.
83. P. A. Hancock, "A Dynamic Model of Stress and Sustained Attention," *Human Factors* 31, no. 5 (1989): 528.
84. Ibid., 519–37.
85. Y. M. Ulrich-Lai and J. P. Herman, "Neural Responses of Endocrine and Autonomic Stress Responses," *Nature Reviews Neuroscience* 10, no. 6 (2009): 397–409.
86. N. Inoue, "Stress and Atherosclerotic Cardiovascular Disease," *Journal of Atherosclerosis and Thrombosis* 21, no. 5 (2014): 391–401.
87. R. von Kanel, "Psychosocial Stress and Cardiovascular Risk—Current Opinion," *Swiss Medical Weekly* 142, no. 0 (2012): w13502.
88. N. Inoue, "Stress and Atherosclerotic Cardiovascular Disease," 394.
89. C. J. Huang, H. E. Webb, M. C. Zourdos et al., "Cardiovascular Reactivity, Stress, and Physical Activity," *Frontiers in Physiology* 4 (2013): 314.
90. M. B. Katan, R. P. Mensink, P. L. Zock, "Trans Fatty Acids and Their Effect on Lipoproteins in Humans," *Annual Review of Nutrition* 15, no. 1 (1995): 473–93.
91. A. Ascherio, M. B. Katan, P. L. Zock et al., "Trans Fatty Acids and Coronary Heart Disease," *New England Journal of Medicine* 340, no. 25 (1999): 1994–98.

92. J. E. Kinsella, G. Bruckner, J. Mai et al., "Metabolism of *Trans* Fatty Acids with Emphasis on the Effects of *Trans, Trans*-octadecadienoate on Lipid Composition, Essential Fatty Acid and Prostaglandins: An Overview," *American Journal of Clinical Nutrition* 34, no. 10 (1981): 2307–18.
93. Z. Y. Chen, G. Pelletier, R. Hollywood et al., "Trans Fatty Acid Isomers in Canadian Human Milk," *Lipids* 30, no. 1 (1995): 15–21.
94. E. Lanque, S. Zamora, and A. Gil, "Dietary Fatty Acids in Early Life: A Review," *Early Human Development* 65, Suppl (2001): S31–41.
95. A. Ascherio, C. H. Hennekens, J. E. Buring et al., "Trans-Fatty Acids Intake and Risk of Myocardial Infarction," *Circulation* 89, no. 1 (1994): 94–101.
96. M. B. Katan, R. Mensink, A. Van Tol et al., "Dietary Trans Fatty Acids and Their Impact on Plasma Lipoproteins," *Canadian Journal of Cardiology* 11, Suppl G (1995): 36G–38G.
97. D. Mozaffarian, M. B. Katan, A. Ascherio et al., "Trans Fatty Acids and Cardiovascular Disease," *New England Journal of Medicine* 13, no. 15 (2006): 1601–13.
98. S. Vega-Lopes, L. M. Ausman, S. M. Jalbert et al., "Palm and Partially Hydrogenated Soybean Oils Adversely Alter Lipoproteins Compared with Canola Oils in Moderately Hyperlipidemic Subjects," *American Journal of Clinical Nutrition* 84, no. 1 (2006): 54–62.
99. R. Micha and D. Mozaffarian, "Trans Fatty Acids: Effects on Cardiometabolic Health and Implications for Policy," *Prostaglandins, Leukotrienes and Essential Fatty Acids* 79, no. 3 (2008): 147–152.
100. R. H. Lustig, "Fructose: It's Alcohol without the Buzz," *Advances in Nutrition an International Review Journal* 4, no. 2 (2013): 226–35.

101. L. Tappy and K. Le, "Metabolic Effects of Fructose and the Worldwide Increase in Obesity," *Physiological Reviews* 90, no. 1 (2010): 23–46.
102. J. D. McPherson, B. H. Shilton, and D. J. Walton, "Role of Fructose in Glycation and Cross-Linking of Proteins," *Biochemistry* 27, no. 6 (1988): 1901–07.
103. A. R. Gaby, "Adverse Effects of Dietary Fructose," *Alternative Medicine Review* 10, no. 4 (2005): 294–306.
104. B. V. Howard and J. Wylie-Rosett, "Sugar and Cardiovascular Disease: A Statement for Healthcare Professionals from the Committee on Nutrition of the Council of Nutrition, Physical Activity, and Metabolism of the American Heart Association," *Circulation* 106, no. 4 (2002): 523–27.
105. 105 . A. Cerami, H. Vlassara, and M. Brownlee, "Protein Glycosylation and the Pathogenesis of Atherosclerosis," *Metabolism* 34, no. 12 (1985): 37–42.
106. T. J. Lyons, "Glycation and Oxidation: A Role in the Pathogenesis of Atherosclerosis," *American Journal of Cardiology* 71, no. 6 (1993): B26–B31.
107. R. K. Johnson, L. J. Appel, M. Brans et al., "Dietary Sugars Intake and Cardiovascular Disease. A Scientific Statement from the American Heart Association," *Circulation* 120, no. 11 (2009): 1011–20.
108. C. M. Brown, A. G. Dulloo, and J. P. Montani, "Sugary Drinks in the Pathogenesis of Obesity and Cardiovascular Diseases," *International Journal of Obesity* 32 (2008): S28–S34.
109. T. T. Fung, V. Malik, K. M. Rexrode et al., "Sweetened Beverage Consumption and Risk of Coronary Heart Disease in Women," *American Journal of Nutrition* 89, no. 4 (2009): 1037–42.

110. V. S. Malik, B. M. Popkin, G. A. Bray et al., "Sugar-Sweetened Beverages, Obesity, Type 2 Diabetes Mellitus, and Cardiovascular Disease Risk," *Circulation* 121, no. 11 (2010): 1356–64.
111. L. de Koning, V. S. Malik, M. D. Kellogg et al., "Sweetened Beverage Consumption, Incident Coronary Heart Disease and Biomarkers of Risk in Men," *Circulation* 125, no. 14 (2012): 1735–41.
112. P. A. James, S. Opanil, B. L. Carter et al., "2014 Evidence-Based Guideline for the Management of High Blood Pressure in Adults. Report from the Panel Members Appointed to the Eight Joint National Committee (JNC 8)," *Journal of the American Medical Association* 311, no. 5 (2014): 507–20.
113. G. Mancia, M. Bombelli, G. Seravalle et al., "Diagnosis and Management of Patients with White-Coat and Masked Hypertension," *Nature Reviews Cardiology* 8, no. 12 (2011): 686–93.
114. B. Cobos, K. Haskard-Zolnierek, and K. Howard, "White Coat Hypertension: Improving the Patient-Health Care Practitioner Relationship," *Psychology Research and Behavior Management* 8 (2015): 133–41.
115. H. Bloch, "Solartherapy, Heliotherapy, Phototherapy, and Biologic Effects: A Historical Overview," *Journal of the National Medical Association* 82, no. 7 (1990): 517–21.
116. F. Nightingale, *Notes on Nursing: What It Is and What It Is Not*, First American Edition (New York: D. Appleton and Company, 1860), 48.
117. R. W. Chesney, "Theobald Palm and his Remarkable Observation: How the Sunshine Vitamin Came to Be Recognized," *Nutrients* 4, no. 1 (2012): 42–51.
118. A. Rollier, "The Construction of an Institution for Heliotherapic Treatment of Surgical Tuberculosis," *Tubercle* 2, no. 6 (1921): 241–50.

119. L. Y. Matsuoka, J. Wortsmand, J. A. MacLaughlin et al., "Sunscreens Suppress Cutaneous Vitamin D3 Synthesis," *Journal of Clinical Endocrinology and Metabolism* 64, no. 6 (1987): 1165–68.
120. A. Faurschou, D. M. Beyer, A. Schmedes et al., "The Relation between Sunscreen Layer Thickness and Vitamin Production after Ultraviolet B Exposure: A Randomized Clinical Trial," *British Journal of Dermatology* 167, no. 2 (2012): 391–95.
121. M. Ramirez-Vick, L. Hernandez-Davila, N. Rodriguez-Rivera et al., "Prevalence of Vitamin D Insufficiency and Deficiency among Young Physicians at University District Hospital in San Juan, Puerto Rico," *Puerto Rico Health Sciences Journal* 34, no. 2 (2015): 83–88.
122. M. F. Holick, "Vitamin D: Importance in Prevention of Cancers, Type 1 Diabetes, Heart Disease and Osteoporosis," *American Journal of Clinical Nutrition* 79, no. 3 (2004): 362–71.
123. M. F. Holick, "Vitamin D Deficiency," *New England Journal of Medicine* 357, no. 3 (2007): 266–81.
124. M. F. Holick, "The D-lightful Vitamin D for Child Health," *Journal of Parenteral and Enteral Nutrition* 36, no. 1 Suppl (2012): 9S–19S.
125. S. Nagapal, S. Na, and R. Rathnachalam, "Noncalcemic Actions of Vitamin D Receptor Ligands," *Endocrine Reviews* 26, no. 5 (2005): 662–87.
126. A. Hossein-Nezhad, A. Spira, and M. F. Hollick, "Influence of Vitamin D Status and Vitamin D3 Supplementation on Genome Wide Expression of White Blood Cells: A Randomized Double-Blind Clinical Trial," *PLOS ONE* 8 (2013): e58725.
127. T. J. Wang, M. J. Pencina, S. L. Booth et al., "Vitamin D Deficiency and Risk of Cardiovascular Disease," *Circulation* 117, no. 4 (2008): 503–11.

128. Abu el Maaty and M. Z. Gad, "Vitamin D Deficiency and Cardiovascular Disease: Potential Mechanisms and Novel Perspectives," *Journal of Nutritional Science and Vitaminology* 59, no. 6 (2013): 479–88.
129. E. Kassi, C. Adampoulos, E. K. Basdra et al., "Role of Vitamin D in Atherosclerosis," *Circulation* 128, no. 23 (2013): 2517–31.
130. P. E. Norman and J. T. Powell, "Vitamin D and Cardiovascular Disease," *Circulation Research* 114, no. 2 (2014): 370–93.
131. I. Mozos and O. Marginean, "Links between Vitamin D Deficiency and Cardiovascular Disease," *BioMed Research International* 2015 (2015): 109275.
132. N. R. Mandarino, F. D. C. M. Junior, J. V. L. Salgado et al., "Is Vitamin D Deficiency a New Risk Factor for Cardiovascular Disease?" *Open Cardiovascular Medicine Journal* 9 (2015): 40–49.
133. M. F. Holick, N. C. Binkley, H. A. Bischoff-Ferrari et al., "Evaluation, Treatment, and Prevention of Vitamin D Deficiency: An Endocrine Society Clinical Practice Guideline," *Journal of Clinical Endocrinology and Metabolism* 96, no. 7 (2011): 1911–30.
134. L. J. Epstein, D. Kristo, P. J. Strollo et al., "Clinical Guideline for Evaluation, Management and Long-Term Care of Obstructive Sleep Apnea in Adults," *Journal of Clinical Sleep Medicine* 5, no. 3 (2009): 263–76.
135. S. M. Shamsuzzaman, B. J. Gersh, and V. K. Somers, "Obstructive Sleep Apnea: Implications for Cardiovascular Disease," *Journal of the American Medical Association* 290, no. 14 (2003): 1906–14.
136. V. K. Kapur, "Obstructive Sleep Apnea: Diagnosis, Epidemiology, and Economics," *Respiratory Care* 55, no. 9 (2010): 1155–64.

137. L. Lavie, "Oxidative Stress Inflammation and Endothelial Dysfunction in Obstructive Sleep Apnea," *Frontiers in Bioscience (Elite Ed.)* 4 (2012): 1391–403.
138. M. Badran, N. Ayas, and I. Laher, "Cardiovascular Complications of Sleep Apnea: Role of Oxidative Stress," *Oxidative Medicine and Cell Longevity* 2014 (2014): 985258.
139. R. Alvarez-Sala, F. Garcia-Rio, F. Del Campo et al., "Sleep Apnea and Cardiovascular Diseases," *Pulmonary Medicine* 2014 (2014): 690273.
140. J. F. Garvey, M. F. Pengo, P. Drakatos et al., "Epidemiological Aspects of Obstructive Sleep Apnea," *Journal of Thoracic Disease* 7, no. 5 (2015): 920–29.
141. B. B. Adhyaru and T. A. Jacobsen, "New Cholesterol Guidelines for the Management of Atherosclerotic Cardiovascular Disease Risk: A Comparison of the 2013 American College of Cardiology/American Heart Association Cholesterol Guidelines with the 2014 National Lipid Association Recommendations for Patient-Centered Management of Dyslipidemia," *Cardiology Clinics* 33, no. 2 (2015): 181–96.
142. H. E. Bays, P. H. Jones, W. V. Brown et al., "National Lipid Association Annual Summary of Clinical Lipidology 2015," *Journal of Clinical Lipidology* 8, no. 6 (2014): S1–36.
143. R. Chou, "Cardiac Screening with Electrocardiography, Stress Echocardiography, or Myocardial Perfusion Imaging: Advice for High-Value Care from the American College of Physicians Cardiac Screening in Low Risk Adults," *Annals of Internal Medicine* 162, no. 6 (2015): 438–47.
144. E. Di Angelantonio, P. Gao, H. Khan et al., "Glycated Hemoglobin Measurement and Prediction of Cardiovascular Disease," *Journal of the American Medical Association* 311, no. 12 (2014): 1225–33.

145. J. K. Pai, L. E. Cahill, F. B. Hu et al., "Hemoglobin A1c is Associated with Increased Risk of Incident Coronary Heart Disease among Apparently Healthy, Nondiabetic Men and Women," *Journal of the American Heart Association* 2, no. 2 (2013): e000077.
146. R. McPherson, J. Frohlich, G. Fodor et al., "Canadian Cardiovascular Society Position Statement—Recommendations for the Diagnosis and Treatment of Dyslipidemia and Prevention of Cardiovascular Disease," *Canadian Journal of Cardiology* 22, no. 11 (2006): 913–27.
147. O. Yousuf, B. D. Mohanty, S. S. Martin et al., "High-Sensitivity C-Reactive Protein and Cardiovascular Disease: A Resolute Belief or an Elusive Link?" *Journal of the American College of Cardiology* 62, no. 5 (2013): 397–408.
148. D. I. Buckley, R. Fu, M. Freeman et al., "C-Reactive Protein as a Risk Factor for Coronary Heart Disease: A Systematic Review and Meta-analyses for the US Preventive Services Task Force," *Annals of Internal Medicine* 151, no. 7 (2009): 483–95.
149. P. M. Ridker, "Clinical Application of C-Reactive Protein for Cardiovascular Disease Detection and Prevention," *Circulation* 107, no. 3 (2003): 363–69.
150. K. H. Bonaa, I. Njolstad, P. M. Ueland et al., "Homocysteine Lowering and Cardiovascular Events after Acute Myocardial Infarction," *New England Journal of Medicine* 354, no. 15 (2006): 1578–88.
151. E. Lonn, S. Yusuf, M. J. Arnold et al., "Homocysteine Lowering with Folic Acid and B Vitamins in Vascular Disease," *New England Journal of Medicine* 354, no. 15 (2006): 1567–77.
152. X. Wang, X. Qin, H. Demirtas et al., "Efficacy of Folic Acid Supplementation in Stroke Prevention: A Meta-analysis," *Lancet* 369, no. 9576 (2007): 1876–82.

153. M. Lee, K. S. Hong, S. C. Chang et al., "Efficacy of Homocysteine-Lowering Therapy with Folic Acid in Stroke Prevention: A Meta-analysis," *Stoke* 41, no. 6 (2010): 1205–12.
154. T. J. Wang, "Vitamin D and Cardiovascular Disease," *Annual Review of Medicine* 67 (2016): 261–72.
155. C. C. Gibson, C. T. Davis, W. Zhu et al., "Dietary Vitamin D and Its Metabolites Non-genomically Stabilize the Endothelium," *PLOS ONE* 10, no. 10 (October 2015): e0140370.
156. R. B. Weller, "Sunlight Has Cardiovascular Benefits Independently of Vitamin D," *Blood Purification* 41, no. 1–3 (2016): 130–34.
157. M. Blaha, M. J. Budoff, L. J. Shaw et al., "Absence of Coronary Artery Calcification and All-Cause Mortality," *Journal of the American College of Cardiology Cardiovascular Imaging* 2, no. 6 (2009): 692–700.
158. K. Nasir, J. Rubin, M. J. Blaha et al., "Interplay of Coronary Artery Calcification and Traditional Risk Factors for the Prediction of All-Cause Mortality in Asymptomatic Individuals," *Circulation: Cardiovascular Imaging* 5, no. 4 (2012): 467–73.
159. R. Nakanishi, D. Li, M. J. Blaha et al., "All-Cause Mortality by Age and Gender Based on Coronary Artery Calcium Scores," *European Heart Journal—Cardiovascular Imaging* (December 24, 2015) PII: jev328. [Epub ahead of print.]
160. I. Zeb and M. Budoff, "Coronary Artery Calcium Screening: Does It Perform Better than Other Cardiovascular Risk Stratification Tools?" *International Journal of Molecular Science* 16, no. 3 (March 23, 2015): 6606–20.
161. P. Greenland, J. S. Alpert, G. A. Belier et al., "2010 ACCF/AHA Guideline for Assessment of Cardiovascular Risk in Asymptomatic Adults: A Report of the American College of Cardiology Foundation/American Heart Association Task Force on Practice

Guidelines," *Journal of the American College of Cardiology* 56, no. 25 (2010): e50–103.

162. H. Korkmaz and O. Onalan, "Evaluation of Endothelial Dysfunction: Flow-Mediated Dilatation," *Endothelium* 15, no. 4 (2008): 157–63.

163. R. M. Bruno, T. Gori, and L. Ghiadoni, "Endothelial Function Testing and Cardiovascular Disease: Focus on Peripheral Arterial Tonometry," *Vascular Health Risk Management* 10 (2014): 577–84.

164. F. G. Fowkes, G. D. Murray, I Butcher et al., "Ankle Brachial Index Combined with Framingham Risk Score to Predict Cardiovascular Events and Mortality: A Meta-Analysis," *Journal of the American Medical Association* 300, no. 2 (2008): 197–208.

165. D. J. Rader, "Human Genetics of Atherothrombotic Disease and Its Risk Factors," *Arteriosclerosis, Thrombosis, and Vascular Biology* 35, no. 4 (2015): 741–47.

166. A. L. Cirino and C. Y. Ho, "Genetic Testing for Inherited Heart Disease," *Circulation* 128, no. 1 (2013): e4–e8.

Proof

Made in the USA
Charleston, SC
22 June 2016